GESELL INSTITUTE OF CHILD DEVELOPMENT

310 Prospect Street
New Haven, Connecticut 06511

"The Children's Doctor" by Dr. Lendon H. Smith is a book that no new mother should be without. It tells her what she needs to know.

The role of the pediatrician, and what he can do for his patients, is changing rapidly and Dr. Smith is in the forefront of this change. It's fair to say that Dr. Arnold Gesell's dream—that it is the doctor's responsibility to advise about age changes in behavior as well as about disease—is fulfilled in this remarkably practical, useful and imaginative book.

Every page contains some bit of helpful, amusing or downright essential information, and the "Quick Reference Directory" is best of all in its crisp, clear explanations of symptoms, diseases and kinds of behavior a new parent wants to know about.

Parents are lucky to be living in a time when there are pediatricians who not only protect and predict but even philosophize about the child's behavior. Dr. Smith is a master at all three.

(Mrs.) Louise Bates Ames
Associate Director

the children's doctor

the children's doctor

by
Lendon Smith, M.D.

Prentice-Hall, Inc., Englewood Cliffs, New Jersey

Cover Photography by John A. Brockway

The Children's Doctor by Lendon Smith, M.D.

Library of Congress Catalog Card Number: 72-77666

Printed in the United States of America • *T*
13-132191-9

0-13-131904-3 pbk.

Prentice-Hall International, Inc., London
Prentice-Hall of Australia, Pty. Ltd., Sydney
Prentice-Hall of Canada, Ltd., Toronto
Prentice-Hall of India Private, Ltd., New Delhi
Prentice-Hall of Japan, Inc., Tokyo

10 9 8 7 6

To the mothers whose trust and
information enabled me to write this book—
one of whom, incidentally, is my wife.

My deep gratitude to Mrs. Peggy Moss for typing and for mending my split infinitives; and also to Mrs. Nancy Elsner for catching my punctuation.

contents

1 ◆◆◆◆◆

INTRODUCTION: THE ROOT OF ALL EVIL

"Do you think it's too early to send him to a psychiatrist?"

Cheerfulness, optimism, and social awareness are valuable assets for almost any career. Combined with a love of children and medical training, these qualities should produce the perfect pediatrician. My father was a wise, kind man who had these traits and became a children's doctor, perhaps because his obvious talents allowed him no other comfortable choice. I recently learned from his cousin that our family of Smiths were all like this.

In his office, my father reassured mothers and comforted sick children, and was still able to be warm and genuine at home. He loved to make people happy; he could make a child feel as though he were the most important person he had seen that day. I have never heard anything derogatory about him.

I think that everyone should have a father like him, although he did make teen-age rebellion difficult. Finding neither hypocrisy to expose nor medieval attitude to deride, I finally singled out one of his cherished views for attack. He believed that a child's personality is established at birth, either through genetic, prenatal, or birth influences, and that environment has relatively little influence.

I had done just enough reading in Freudian psychology to see that environment was the *whole* answer to psychic development; anybody with reasonable potential would develop according to his surroundings. (For example, my mother had toilet-trained me early, so I was obsessive-compulsive in my desire to perform successfully.) If the environmental influences were good, he would be a good person; if bad, he would be bad, QED. I could not see how heredity could possibly be the key to personality development.

Once, during the time that my father was the medical director of a foundling home, he conducted a little experiment of his own. (He did not publish the results, of course, because he did not think they were sufficiently valuable.) He picked out twelve children, all of them eighteen months old, who had been in the same nursery since birth. All were reasonably healthy and of about the same size and weight. He put them together in one room and gave each child a little box to play with. He left them there for thirty or forty-five minutes with no adult supervision, and at the end of that time he returned to record the results.

One child was in a corner hugging twelve little boxes. Three children were fighting to get their boxes back, two others had gone to sleep, three were crying, one was sucking his thumb, one was examining a piece of string he had found, and the last was picking lint out of his navel. Each child (so my father explained) was behaving in a way that expressed his own personality. Here with the twelve boxes was the type who had to have everything— an aggressive, mean bully, like Hitler. The three trying to get their boxes back showed they had a certain amount of strength and fight; they were trying to recover what was rightfully theirs. The others had sour-graped the whole situation, figuring "what's the point?" or else were seeking to cope with their anger by crying or lint-picking.

My father was convinced his experiment clearly demonstrated his old belief that hereditary or genetic influences will determine the personality. The one who had swiped all the boxes would grow up to be mean and aggressive, running roughshod over others. As they matured, the other children would also retain their individual reactions to frustration—sour grapes, somnolence, tears, or retreat to oral gratification. Genetic influences were the only variables my father could see, because he was sure that the environment had been the same for each child since birth.

"Not so!" I countered. With great sophistry, I pointed out the amateurishness of his experiment. How could he possibly control all the variables in the surroundings and care of these babies? Maybe one got changed or fed sooner because his cry was especially irritating to the nurse. Maybe one was cuter and got extra cuddling. Perhaps another had colic and had to be picked up more. Father muttered something about the lack of respect young people were showing their elders these days, and we went our ways, neither of us having convinced the other of anything— except that one generation does not always communicate well with the next one.

I must have outgrown my desire to rebel, because I too became a doctor and then a pediatrician. But I was still convinced that every baby was born "decent and worthwhile" and that any neurosis was the fault of parental attitudes. "Straighten out the next generation all over the world," I thought, "and psychoses, crime, and wars will disappear." How perfect to dedicate myself to pediatrics, where I could influence a family from birth on! I was so normal that I would easily persuade mothers to adopt my values and thus stem the neurotic tide.

As my family grew along with my practice, a few roadblocks began to slow down my journey to worldwide psychic utopia. I actually began to wonder if other factors might be operative besides environment. For instance, once you have observed a few newborn babies it becomes quite obvious that each has a different activity level. "There are race horses and plug horses," as my father used to say. As a "race horse" grows up, he maintains his basic trait and is often accident prone, impulsive, and touchy. A "plug horse" is passive, responds less to pain, and is more likely to be a spectator.

Twins have the same environment. If behavior is dissimilar in identical twins, the explanation must be a difference in birth experiences; differences in fraternal twins can be explained by genetic factors. How does a boy with six older sisters and an absent father know he is a boy? Why the different personalities in a large family with the same parents, similar environment, and identical love and discipline? Why is one such a black sheep?

Did the mother pick him out at birth and say, "I think I'll turn this kid into a real mess"?

Most of the mothers who came to see me were anxious to rear their children properly. They were conscientious and seemed to know instinctively how to provide a "home." They wanted reassurance and encouragement. I had a rule—and still do—that if I am comfortable talking to them, they are normal mothers. Many of these normal women told me about rotten behavior in their children. How could these good mothers have sabotaged their children's emotions? Was my intuition wrong? Was my training faulty? Was my father right?

I began to wonder about a few of my *own* cherished views. And I finally abandoned my adolescent naiveté when the personalities of my own children began to emerge, each of the five showing different traits. Why does one of my sons resemble and act so like my father that I can almost believe he is reincarnated? Why does one of my daughters wiggle her finger like my mother does unless there is a gene for finger-wiggling? (If this had been environmentally produced, my wife would have put a stop to it long ago because she cannot stand finger-wiggling.) Does our pouting child pout because of maternal rejection? Or could it be his chromosomes carry a paternal gene for pouting?

These observations forced me to adopt a new theory of personality development. My thesis now is that if you have provided the standard love and limits and you still have a black sheep in your family, the trouble may well lie within the child and his genetic background. Or he may have some subtle neurological hurt, or an allergy may make him irritable, or any number of rarely recognized entities may make him surly, mean, or at least difficult or different. The point is, the root of the evil may be biological rather than psychological. If blue eyes, blond hair, and facial features are inheritable, then why is it so far-fetched that behavior traits, thumb-sucking, bed-wetting, and a host of other so-called psychological problems are genetically determined?

In other words, possibly your impossible, ornery, stubborn, irritable child has *inherited* all the wrong genes (from the other side of the family, of course). Nevertheless, friends, neighbors, and a host of women's magazines will tell you that parents—and especially you, the mother—have wrecked your child's psyche by postnatal influences. Thinly veiled denunciations of your mothering ability most frequently come from your mother-in-law. After all, she did a great job of rearing *her* son or you would not have married him. Therefore, rather than quit while she is ahead, she will be happy to oversee the rearing of her grandchildren, too. And if their behavior is not ideal, it must be your fault.

The guilty mother usually feels psychotherapy is the only answer; the psychiatrist reinforces this feeling by finding some twisted attitude in the home. How could it have happened? She studied psychology in school; she read the magazines; she listened to experts.

Where did the mother go wrong? She wanted him at conception, she loved him when he arrived, she enjoyed feeding him when he was hungry, she soothed him when he cried, she reassured him when he was afraid, she dressed him in cute clothes with money she could have spent on herself. She took him to the doctor for checkups and shots, she sent him to the best nursery school, and what good did it all do? He is an emotional cripple. She tries to love him, but she is getting to hate him.

I feel a mother often overreacts to difficult behavior that is physiologically caused, and that *then* the psychological factors become superimposed. After all, how awful do you have to be to wreck a little child's psyche? We have all seen those terrible homes down the street where the parents drink and fight all the time, or are extremely rigid, punitive, or permissive. In these cases, we assume the children will be emotionally twisted, but frequently the youngsters grow up to be reasonably normal adults.

Some years ago, I was called to see a young mother who had just had her first baby. Apparently conception was no problem—she sailed through that without a sign of trauma. But she felt that the care and feeding was going to be too much. I saw her in the hospital when the baby was but a few hours old, and she seemed rife with anxieties about her abilities as a mother. She had never changed or fed a baby, so I had to teach her about bathing, changing (even folding) the diapers, feeding—everything that we have often assumed women know instinctively. As I was doing all this, I thought what a perfect setup this was to produce a colicky baby. If any mother was going to transmit her tensions to her baby, this was the one.

I rushed back to the office to await the hourly phone calls from her, but none came. I became engrossed in my daily practice and figured she had gone to someone else because she had found out I was taking Wednesday afternoons off. Imagine my surprise when, after a month, she brought her pink, fat, healthy baby in for his first checkup. "No problem," she effused, "I just fed and changed him, and he ate and slept." Some luck, I thought. I am sure that if that baby had gone "peep" at the wrong time the mother would have lost what little confidence she had, and would have become so nervous and distraught that the whole house would have been in an uproar. The child kept his mouth shut almost as if he knew what might have happened to him. He continued to do well and is now a normal, rebellious adolescent. Encouraged by her success, the mother tried it again, and is now rearing a fine girl.

Another mother had a baby and invited me to check him out. "Everything is fine," I told her after the examination.

"Sorry to have bothered you with my fifth one," she said happily. "I just wanted to know if he had all his equipment. I'll nurse him, of course, and come in later for the shots." She was a jolly, secure mother who felt comfortable in her role.

Here's the kicker, though. Ten days later she called in tears because her baby was screaming night and day with gas and colic. She had lost her old confidence; she felt completely inadequate, and her household had gone to pot. Actually, the baby was allergic to the cow's milk his mother was drinking. We stopped the milk and soon got the family back in one piece again.

This is a good illustration of how a child can stir up problems. If the problems are not solved, modified, or at least recognized for what they are, then parents (and more especially mothers) react to the child and his symptoms with worry and confusion. If prolonged, a mother's attitude alone will initiate psychiatric problems. Many mothers get tense and edgy when saddled with a baby who has an allergy. For months they have to hold, rock, and mop up after him during the day, and sit up at night trying to comfort him. The normal mother still loves her fussy child, but she does have to make a special effort to *like* him all the time.

A sickly child who needs expensive medicine can run up a whopping bill at the drug store; a normal mother will not begrudge this, but even the most unselfish homemaker cannot help but get rankled when subtracting outgo from income. A casual observer sees only the overall nervous tension in the home and assumes that the mother was the instigator of it all, because she is the one doing all the complaining. The observer forgets one thing—the mother was fun-loving, happy, and relaxed before the baby came to foul up the picture. The point is that it is often the child who ties the family into an all-entwining, self-perpetuating, psychopathic Gordian knot.

But if terrible behavior can derive from genes or neurological or constitutional predispositions, does that imply it is fixed and nontreatable? Definitely not. New techniques of modifying symptoms and behavior (with and without drugs) are now effective in a high percentage of patients.

The pediatrician should play the key role in organizing the treatment program. He can help support a mother's flagging spirit by showing her that her child's problems are not always her fault, by warning her about the different crochety phases a child goes through, and by breaking the vicious cycles that lead to psychiatric sickness. And a pediatrician's book can help her rear her child, help her accept her child's idiosyncrasies, and help her develop proper attitudes, thus preventing *secondary* psychological problems.

The role of the pediatrician has gradually changed from what it was a generation ago. Thirty to forty years ago, my father's job was fairly clear-cut: He had to check diarrhea, watch out for diphtheria, and reassure parents that doctors were doing everything possible for pneumonia, measles, scarlet fever, and the many terrible infectious diseases that raged before the days of antibiotics. He went on many house calls and practiced much art with his science.

The "new" child-care specialist may spend less time on health and nutritional maintenance, and more time on the behavioral and emotional aspects of his patients. The frequent checkups we suggest in the early months and years of life are designed not only to assure immunization shots, good growth, and nutrition, but also to ferret out signs of incipient emotional problems in the child and to correct abnormal parental traits, attitudes, and ideas.

All pediatricians, whether we know it or not, practice preventive psychiatry.

In one sense, the pediatrician acts as an educator. He teaches the mother what is normal for her child in growth and development, and he trains her to spot trouble early, when it is much easier to reverse a bad trend. The doctor wants her to develop an attitude of casual concern; if *her* mother was responsible and mature, she probably will be so, too. But if the mother is less than perfect, sometimes—I said *sometimes*—the doctor can still support her waning psyche and train her to be a reasonably good mother.

After I had been in practice a few years, I noticed the great number of problems—physical or developmental in origin—that mothers were dealing with as if they were emotional.

At the age of two years, two things happen to a child almost at the same time. His mother tries to toilet-train him, and he loses his appetite because his rate of growth has been slowed. He is normally somewhat hostile and stubborn at this age, and if he suspects that he's about to do something his mother wants him to do, he will say, "No!" This is his favorite word. He will stiffen and cry when placed on the potty, as if he knew that to relax and smile might empty his rectum, and *that* would be collaborating with the enemy. He decides never to have another bowel movement for the rest of his life, so he holds it until it gets big and hard and needs to be delivered by suppositories or enemas. This treatment frequently causes pain and spasm in the anal area and reaffirms his previous conviction of "never again." The battle continues, with mother and child fighting over this worthless bit of waste as if it were gold.

But this is not the only battlefront. While the mother is trying to "get" at the nether end, she is trying to "give" at the near end. A year earlier her child had been gaining a pound or two a month; now he gains a pound or two in six months and, of course, needs less food. One poor meal a day seems plenty for most children two to four years of age, but when the mother does not know this, she continues to serve overly generous portions. When the child comes to the table, his throat is dry from the frequent crying and whining characteristic of that age, so he selects the foods that slide down most easily—white foods (carbohydrates, starches, bananas, rice, etc.) and dairy products.

These, of course, are terribly constipating and only serve to aggravate the bowel problem.

If these two areas of conflict do not lead to daily tears and screaming on both sides, there are two more hassles that will. At about age two a child is cutting some big molars, which makes him surly. This is bad enough. And if he continues his iron-poor, white-food diet, he can become rather severely anemic. This further reduces his appetite for the very foods (meat and fruit) that might correct his anemia as well as soften his stools. These interrelated miseries, plus the trials of eating and eliminating, add up to four potential areas of conflict.

Only rarely do pediatricians see this convoluted psychosomatic mess in patients who have been coming for regular visits since birth. We are usually able to warn the mother about the next approaching phase of growth, and thus help her anticipate the problems which may occur. If such difficulties are allowed to develop, they can take months to relieve and still leave psychic scars.

The distractible school-aged child—who has a short attention span and cannot stay in his seat—illustrates the result of a neurologically based problem unresolved at an earlier age. The teacher blames the mother for not teaching him "self-control." The mother has tried bribery, severe discipline, and deprivation, but nothing works. Today, the pediatrician knows the diagnosis is the "hypermotor condition" and can control the situation with drugs. He can sometimes detect the first signs of this problem in the early weeks and months of life, prepare the mother for the teacher's reproaches, and even forestall them.

The child who awakens at night is often thought to be insecure, but wakefulness is more likely to be due to pinworms.

Headaches may certainly be due to some suppressed hostility, but not infrequently they indicate a food allergy.

The child who wets the bed every night may very well have an emotional problem, but he may have an allergy or be such a sound sleeper that his lazy brain doesn't know what his busy bladder is doing.

The mean child who elbows his way through life possibly may have learned this from mean, punitive parents. He may also be suffering from some hyperactive electrical "short circuit" in his brain.

These are actually very common conditions a doctor meets frequently in daily practice. But because there are few obvious clues or tests with which to diagnose them, the doctor has to be always suspicious. Sometimes he can only diagnose them by treating them. For example, if a child is treated for worms and after three days of treatment he begins to sleep through the night, his sleeplessness was probably due to worms and not anxiety. Again, if the symptom is allowed to go untreated, the reaction it produces can lead to a psychiatric problem throughout the family.

The problem of the irritable, irritating child must occur in up to 20 percent of all households. Child-care specialists and general practitioners know that a good number of adults are neurotic, psychotic, or unstable enough to make poor parents. The problem is compounded, of course, if a touchy child comes into a touchy home. At the present time, no one has advocated (out loud, at least) eugenic laws that would require psychiatric clearance for couples before they can mate. So we will continue to need pediatricians—*and* child psychologists and psychiatrists.

I refer plenty of children to psychologists and psychiatrists for testing, evaluation, and treatment, but before the referral is made, I want to be reasonably sure I haven't overlooked an organic cause.

If you are living with a child whose behavior drives you up the wall, is it cheating to treat him with a medicine that alters his behavior? Psychiatrists would have us believe that it is dangerous to treat *symptoms* and not root out causes. But if an errant gene was responsible for an irritable bioelectrical focus deep in the thalamus of the brain where neurology and psychiatry interwine, what can be prescribed? A new head? Pharmacological research will soon have some answers, and drugs will eventually become more specific in their application. Most parents are reluctant to use medication for behavior control, but when the case is severe, I feel drugs are as appropriate as penicillin for strep throat or insulin for diabetes.

Frequently a mother wants *something* done before her home breaks up because of the child's antics. Often we treat her disagreeable child with medicine. In more than 50 to 70 percent of cases, behavior improves. In private practice it is hard to know how much benefit occurs simply because the mother knows something is being done. Could a sugar pill have been just as effective? In any event, improvement is noted. This gives the family a chance to examine and alter their attitudes under the doctor's guidance. Rewards for *acceptable* behavior can be substituted for punishment for negative behavior. The child begins to see, "If I act this way, the world acts better to me." He is getting positive feedback. And if the home is reasonably well balanced—or has improved because *he* has improved—then the new, better family interaction will be permanent and the medicine can be discontinued. Thus both child and environment have to change. Medicine can be used to control a child while therapy is being given, and in many cases the medicine is the therapy. Treatment is more successful in a child because of his brain's great potential for spontaneous improvement. It is as if the drug allows the nervous system to try newer, more socially acceptable habit patterns—which then become a fixed part of the personality because the environment reinforced them.

This book, I hope, will help you recognize deviations from normal behavior. By indicating what to expect at different ages, I hope to relieve fears and feelings of inadequacy and make you confident as a parent. I would like you to feel less guilty if you sometimes resent your child's behavior.

I will try to explain the differences and interrelationships between physical and psychological illness. You should learn how to deal with some of the annoying—but trivial—childhood complaints and decide which you can handle, which are for the doctor, and which are for the teacher.

Chances are, you are already doing a lot better than you think in guiding your child to maturity. Cheerful optimism and a sense of humor will help in your child-rearing adventure, and some of these traits should rub off on your child before you push him out of the nest

2 ◆◆—◆—◆◆

THE FIRST MONTHS OF FEEDING

"He can't be hungry; he just ate!"

Most authorities agree that you should feed your baby when he's hungry. This seems to make so much sense that it's hardly worth mentioning. A normal seven-pound new baby who is reasonably awake and alert needs from fourteen to twenty ounces of milk every twenty-four hours. If there are about twenty calories per ounce in the milk that you are feeding him, he should get at least two ounces for each pound he weighs. A baby on milk can empty his stomach in just an hour and a half, so if you can feed a new baby every hour and a half or two hours, he will get his nutritional quota during his twelve waking hours and may possibly sleep all night long. If he can take two ounces eight times a day, he is going to get enough to take care of his needs.

If he's growing at a terrific rate or he's very active, then you may have to give him more because his hunger will undoubtedly be greater. A baby destined to be a small adult can get all his calories during his twelve waking hours and not have to wake up in the night; he is unlikely to eat as much as a baby who will eventually be six feet tall. But if he's active and going to be a good-size adult—if both you and your husband are five feet ten or six feet tall—he won't be able to sleep through the night until he's three or four months old, because he's growing too fast to get all his calories during his twelve waking hours.

In general, the good rule is this: At least two ounces of milk for every pound, over a twenty-four-hour period, for the first three months of life. Milk provides fluid and enough protein, calcium, carbohydrates, and calories to take care of your baby's needs in those first months. If he sleeps for six hours during the day and he's up every couple of hours in the night to make up for it, then you are perfectly justified in waking him up during the *day* to see if you can get him on a better schedule. If you feed him every two or three hours during the day, maybe he will sleep for four, five, or even eight hours at night. Maybe.

Just about any good type of milk (homogenized milk or any of the standard prepared formulas to which you can add water) will provide the necessary twenty calories per ounce. Incidentally, if it is safe for you to drink the water without boiling it, you don't need to boil it for the baby. But if you have any disease or skin infections, or if you are not sure about the water that comes from the well, it's probably better to boil it for ten minutes before using it for the formula. You don't have to boil the bottles if you don't want to. If you use a bottle brush to get the milk curds out, then washing them along with the dishes is good enough.

Despite the beautiful job that the milk-processing people have done to make cow's milk compatible with human infants' stomachs, cow's milk is still best suited for calves. Breast-feeding is an important and desirable method of feeding. However, many mothers feel that it is going to wreck their figure (which is nonsense) and that it ties the mother down (which may or may not be true). In addition to those mothers who don't *want* to, many mothers are *unable* to breast-feed their babies. The real reason may be that most hospitals tend to discourage them. The standard hospital puts the babies in a common nursery and the mothers in separate rooms down the hall. When the baby cries from hunger before the standard four hours are up, the nurse, usually busy with other things, may not be able to drop whatever she's doing and bring this crying baby out to his mother. A feed-on-demand schedule is the best way to get breast-feeding started.

Plentiful statistics indicate that in rooming-in situations, where babies are brought to their mothers shortly after birth (or after she has recovered enough so that she won't drop the poor thing), 85 percent of those who want to nurse are able to do so. In the separate-nursery method in the standard hospital, only 35 percent are successful.

However, there is a growing trend for hospitals to discharge a healthy mother between the second and the fourth day after delivery. This seems rather quick to us old-timers, but it has been found that mother and child stand less of a chance of contracting a hospital-based infection. Doctors find that many mothers recover from childbirth a lot more rapidly if they get out of bed in the first few postnatal days. In other words, don't get pregnant just to get a few days' rest in the hospital—you will only find yourself being kicked out in three days, which is scarcely time enough to get a couple of naps. But if you have some help at home, your early release from the rigidly scheduled hospital will aid breast feeding.

Even if your baby has not had rooming-in conditions, he may be able to nurse successfully because you will be home with him on the third or fourth day when the milk starts to come in. Breast milk in any measurable amount usually is not produced until about the fourth day, but the sucking stimulation necessary for milk production should be started within the first few post-natal hours.

In general, you should breast-feed your baby with this in mind: He can empty his stomach in an hour and a half, so he should be allowed to eat that frequently if he wants. Making him wait for four hours only frustrates both you and him. He may take a couple of sucks and then fall asleep exhausted, not stimulating breast milk to come in an adequate flow. If you have reasonably normal nipples and your baby has a good sucking reflex, perhaps the best way is to give him the breast every hour and a half to three hours during the day. Hopefully, he will get his quota during the twelve daylight hours and then go maybe four, five, or six hours at night. That's the ideal way to feed a baby. Many authorities now feel that if there is any sort of allergy background in your family, you should try to breast-feed your baby, because of the likelihood that he will develop an allergy to cow's milk (which we will discuss later).

There are a few pitfalls to breast-feeding a baby, but if a mother is motivated and determined enough, she is usually successful. Pediatricians and many obstetricians have found that if the mother has to ask the doctor whether or not she should breast-feed, this usually means that she does not want to do so. Our answer is usually another question: "What do *you* want to do?" A lot of psychological motivation is required for successful breast-feeding, and we cannot force it on a mother who has made up her mind that it will not work. Certainly she may have some trouble if she has a bad infection or is exhausted after a very difficult delivery. If her baby is huge, she may not have enough milk to satisfy him, and his hunger cries may make her feel so guilty that she turns to the bottle—for him, that is. The baby gets satisfied from the more plentiful bottle, and this in turn discourages the production of milk. Nursing soon fails.

One drawback of breast-feeding is the slight inconvenience of drippy breasts. Another disadvantage is the fact that the mother must be present at every feeding, and that her husband is unable to help out very much. But the advantages of breast-feeding far outweigh the disadvantages. Even if you are planning to nurse your baby for only the first month or two of life, I feel it is terribly important that you do so.

A very worthwhile breast-feeding organization in the United States is called *La Leche League.* They are almost as gung-ho about their group as Alcoholics Anonymous is about theirs. Advocates of this group in almost every section of the country are more than anxious to help mothers start a successful breast-feeding program. If you are even half-interested in breast-feeding and need a little push from the outside, you might contact this group for some moral support. Most mothers offer one bottle of cow's milk a day, even though it is considered cheating. The milk supply is usually at its lowest between 4 and 8 P.M. Ideally, the husband can give the bottle at this time while mother fixes dinner.

You should continue the prenatal vitamins that you were taking before to keep yourself adequately nourished and of course to pass some extra vitamins on to your baby. Any reasonably good diet, consisting of some animal protein, fruit, vegetables and grain seems to be adequate. Most authorities feel that if you drink a quart of whole milk or skim milk and a quart of some other kind of fluids every day, you will not become dehydrated. Many breast-feeding mothers are desperately hungry and find that they are overeating and gaining a great deal of weight. This may or may not be due to breast-feeding, but it is a complaint so common that it should be considered if you have an obesity problem.

When I do get called by a mother who is successfully breast-feeding her baby, she is usually concerned about the large amount of gas her baby develops. Some things that a mother eats get into her milk and can seriously upset the baby's digestion. A few diet taboos should be observed in the first few few weeks of breast-feeding. The most common offenders are fish—especially tuna fish—garlic, onions, cabbage, and beans. Some mothers find that they cannot eat chocolate because this upsets the baby; others discover they have to cut out citrus fruits and tomatoes because the baby breaks out in a rash. I have also found that corn, pork, wheat, and even eggs can give difficulty.

If you are breast-feeding your baby because of allergies in the family, you may often find you yourself cannot drink any cow's milk, because in essence, your baby then gets cow's milk protein—to which he is allergic—and becomes quite colicky. If a mother of a successfully breast-fed baby stops nursing him because her child is filled with gas and then changes to a cow's-milk formula, the baby's gas is then even worse. But by the time she finds out the real source of the trouble, her breasts have dried up and it is too late to get the baby back on breast-feeding. If your breast-fed baby has very frothy, gas-filled stools and is very crampy but seems to be getting a proper amount of milk, you should simply look to your diet. Something is fermenting in the baby's intestinal tract, and if he is drinking only your own milk, the problem must be something you are eating.

Many a mother in tears has called me at five o'clock in the afternoon because her otherwise perfect baby has been screaming since two. My first question is, "Is he getting enough milk?" She will say she is sure he is. My second question is, "What did you eat for lunch?" And almost nine times out of ten she had a tuna-fish sandwich. Maybe she even put a little bit of onion in with the tuna fish and this added to the distress.

Once when my wife was nursing our first baby, she had a piece of garlic bread for lunch and nursed the baby afterward. The baby started to scream. Not knowing what terrible intestinal problem our daughter had developed, I rushed home. When I picked the baby up and burped her, I could smell garlic on her breath. It had gone right through the two of them, and I was getting it third-hand.

Sometimes even the vitamins you are taking will have enough fish oils in them to get into your baby and upset him. But after breast-feeding has been well established (and when your baby is sleeping right through the night), you may find you can eat some spicy food that is on the *verboten* list—providing you wait until after the last nursing at night. Hopefully, by the next morning the irritants will be out of your system. But remember, the night you indulge might be just the night that your baby will wake up at one o'clock, and you will have to feed him breast milk that is full of all sorts of garlic and spices and cheese and fish cakes and whatnot. And your baby may just scream from two in the morning until the next afternoon.

The nursing mother's next biggest distress is not knowing how much milk her baby is getting. She can count the ounces when she is bottle-feeding, but with breast-feeding this is not easy to measure. Some mothers weigh their baby before and after nursing to see how many ounces he has taken, but this is difficult with the less-than-optimum home scales. The amount of urine he puts out every day indicates how much milk is going through him; if there's enough fluid, he's getting enough milk. A baby on bottle or breast rarely gains more than an ounce a day, so if you can weigh your baby just once a week and if he has gained at least four ounces, then he is probably getting an adequate supply.

A rather reassuring rule is that if your baby nurses for ten or fifteen minutes and falls off to sleep as if he had gone into a coma, he's probably getting an adequate supply. A hungry baby seldom lets you rest. If he sucks for ten or fifteen minutes and then screams and looks around for more, you will have to assume he did not get enough at that feeding. Then you will have to decide whether to give both breasts at that feeding or whether to supplement with some cow's milk. This may be strictly against the rules, because the real breast-feeding purists believe breast-fed babies should be given no cow's milk whatsoever. Once bottles are started, they soon lead to a downhill course. More and more bottles seem to be needed, until the baby abandons the breast altogether. (It is all right to give a little extra sugar water: one teaspoon of sugar to six ounces of water is fine.)

A mother not used to breast-feeding may be alarmed by her baby's rather distressing stools. He is almost never constipated. His stools are usually the consistency of thick pea soup, quite yellow, with a faint acid or vinegar odor. The smell is rarely offensive, but when solids are started or cow's milk is given, the stools then develop a more disagreeable odor. The totally breast-fed baby has anywhere from three sloppy stools a day to as few as one every five days. (If he has gone that many days, this stool is usually quite explosive, but you should not consider him constipated unless the stool is hard—which is almost never the case.) When breast-feeding is successful, a baby sucks for ten or fifteen minutes, goes off to sleep, wakes up anywhere from one and a half to six hours later, sucks for ten or fifteen minutes, and goes back to sleep. Once every two or three days, he has this large, sloppy stool that really fills his pants down to his knees.

As I have said, there are some disadvantages to breast-feeding, so many people compromise. One hundred percent breast-feeding is rare because prepared milk substitutes are so convenient. Most nursing mothers make some plans for a relief bottle of some weak fluid like skim milk or a watered-down solution of powdered milk. But you will find that unless you introduce this relief bottle during the first month, your baby will refuse to take it thereafter. If you are nearby, he thinks he is being cheated or somehow going to be poisoned by the bottle, and demands the real thing. A stubborn baby seems determined to starve if you try to offer him a bottle. He gets one whiff of the artificial nipple and just turns up his nose and screams for twenty-four hours. He is upset from hunger and frustration, and is showing the first indications of real anger and hostility. But usually the two of you can come to terms, and hunger wins the day.

Many babies get breast milk so rapidly that it almost seems to choke them. They gulp and swallow as if trying to keep from drowning, because the milk is really squirting out of the nipples. Some mothers feel that babies do not get enough sucking pleasure when the milk comes this rapidly, so many give them a pacifier after nursing to help fulfill the sucking drive. The controversy is still on—some purists refuse to have a pacifier around the house because they are such "dirty" things. It depends a lot on individual taste—I personally think that the nipple, when compared to the thumb, is the lesser of two evils. If your baby has a great deal of sucking drive, he is going to find his thumb soon enough, and the nipple would be a more satisfactory substitute.

In our culture, successful breast-feeding is usually continued for a minimum of three months. Many find it so satisfactory to all concerned that they keep it up beyond nine months or even after twelve months, which is the traditional American time to try a baby on the cup. As your baby gets beyond six months and has more solids pushed at him, you may find you can reduce the breast-feedings to two a day. Some mothers who like to breast-feed keep it up even after their children cut some teeth—which you probably would find a discouragement. You may, though, find you can get your ten-month-old, sleep-resistant baby into bed more easily if you lie down with him and nurse him for a few minutes at bedtime. He may be taking the cup all day, but you can soothe him by nursing before his nap or at night.

There is no right or wrong time to stop, and much depends on your own needs and feelings. I understand that in the Orient, perhaps because of sanitation problems, a child will continue to nurse from the mother until he is several years old. This is certainly unusual. Teeth coming in, somewhere between seven and ten months, seem to be Mother Nature's clue that milk is less important and solid foods more so. Milk has almost no iron in it, so even a baby who is drinking nothing but human milk—which is supposed to be ideal for humans—can become anemic. Gradually introducing solid foods after six or seven months will reduce the milk consumption.

Let me reassure mothers who have found it physically, emotionally, or intellectually impossible to breast-feed. Many feel terribly guilty; they feel that somehow they are not good mothers for their babies. They worry that their children may grow up to have some terrible psychological blight because they were not breast-fed. "He didn't get enough warmth and affection, and this will wreck his chances for security." Don't worry: Many studies have tried to relate emotional security to breast-feeding, or neurosis in an adult to bottle-feeding, and all have come to naught. There are many other factors involved in the care, handling, and feeding of a baby. Breast milk, although it is obviously what humans were designed to have, is not so essential that its absence will blight a child's psyche. The fact that you were able to have the child and that you are able to love your child are proofs enough that you are a woman and a mother.

Bottle-feeding attempts to simulate breast-feeding. The mother usually tries to hold and love her baby when she is bottle-feeding, but a goodly number of babies are upset if they are held. It does not mean that there is anything wrong with your baby if he prefers to have the bottle propped. Again, there are those who feel that this is a terrible thing to do to a baby since he won't get all that love and security that he's supposed to have. Some babies just do not want to be touched and handled when they are eating —it is too distracting. I suppose this especially might be true of a nervous baby who is more aware of his environment and easily overstimulated. Many mothers have found that if the bottle is propped, the baby is less likely to spit up the milk; he drinks the milk faster and seems to be more content. The stomach curves from left to right, so if he's fed while lying on his right side, the air bubbles will remain on the top and he's less likely to spit up his milk.

Obviously, the most comfortable way to handle a baby is to cradle him and hold him up next to your breast. You are supposed to sing and talk to your baby, but this should not be too distracting, because he is busy eating. This is the usual picture of motherhood—the warmth, the cradling, the loving, the cooing, and the satisfactory warm milk going down to fill his stomach.

If you are nervous or tense about handling or feeding, you will only transmit this nervousness to your baby. The simple act of holding some touchy babies overexcites them. This, again, does not imply that you are unfit as a mother; only that you need to relax more with the baby and take your time. Propping the bottle is perfectly acceptable. You certainly should not feel guilty if you have the kind of baby that seems to spit up every time you hold him.

It is estimated that about one out of fifteen babies develops some type of milk allergy in the first few weeks of life. That one baby may be getting along very smoothly until about three or four weeks of age—it usually takes that long to develop an allergy to cow's milk—at which time he may have any of the following symptoms. He may be spitting up or vomiting, even to the point that he appears to have an obstruction. He may be full of gas and bloated. He may be screaming, just be unhappy, or fail to gain weight. He may have terribly sloppy, gas-filled stools. His stools may be green all the time (this is bile coloration—his green bile is not getting a chance to change to the normal yellow color). He may break out with eczema, he may develop a terrible red rash around his anal opening. He may have phlegm that sounds like sinus trouble, postnasal drip, or a plugged allergic nose. Or he may actually wheeze as though he has asthma.

All of these symptoms may develop at the same time or singly. The baby may display only one, but if he is uncomfortable enough, you have to change his milk. If it is an allergy, you should see his symptoms improve within twenty-four to forty-eight hours after the change. If they *don't* improve whatsoever after you have taken him off cow's milk and put him on some substitute (such as soy bean milk, or a meat type of milk, or goat's milk), then some other problem is at fault. Sometimes a doctor has to use guesswork to diagnose a baby with a milk allergy. Many babies are treated for what seems to be an obstruction such as pyloric stenosis or an infection, when their problem is really an allergy that is avoided by changing to another type of milk.

I have seen a baby who developed a wheeze and phlegm from cow's milk and who was later put on soy bean milk. The wheeze and phlegm disappeared, but he got diarrhea and gas. When he was changed to goat's milk these symptoms disappeared, but he broke out with severe eczema. In this situation, the mother found that she had to give three or four different milks during the day. In the morning she would give cow's milk, a soy bean milk at noon, goat's milk in the afternoon, and some sort of meat formula in the evening. This way her baby did not get enough of any one milk to produce the major symptoms. He had a few of the symptoms all the time, but not severely enough to make him unhappy. Finally, at the age of eight or ten months, he could tolerate cow's milk. Milk allergies are common enough that if your baby develops any of the above symptoms, it would be worthwhile to experiment with milk changes.

One distressing feature about the artificial milks is that a baby often spits them up. Sometimes it is a fat intolerance—and the baby does better if put on a low-fat diet (such as going from whole milk or 3.8 percent butterfat content to 2 percent or even skim milk). Again, the symptoms should abate immediately, and if they do not, some other technique has to be used.

For lack of a better term, colic is any crying that cannot be related to hunger. There seems to be a wide variety of causes, the most common of which would be a milk allergy. The pediatric textbooks dismiss this distressing condition by stating that it is an overreactive intestinal tract in a baby who is being overstimulated by his environment. This does not help either the pediatrician or the mother who has to live in the same house with all that screaming.

The following possibilities should be considered when dealing with a fussy, crying, unhappy baby:

(1) *Hunger.* If giving him an adequate supply of nourishing milk does not stop your baby's screams his condition is called colic. When you're trying to keep your baby on a schedule, you may feel that he must have colic if he hollers less than four hours after feeding. But if an hour and a half has gone by, your baby's unhappiness is most likely caused by hunger. Babies can be fed every hour and a half during the day, and if they are comfortable and relaxed after each feeding, they do not have colic. However, if he gets an adequate supply of milk and bellows within twenty or thirty minutes, *then* it is probably colic. But if he's fairly comfortable and lets an hour and a half go by, assume that he's hungry.

(2) *Allergy.* This has been discussed previously. If your baby is not suffering from hunger, but is full of gas and seems bloated, you should try changing the milk. If he is better within twenty-four to forty-eight hours after the change and remains so, it implies that he has a milk allergy. If you go back to the original milk and he starts to scream with gas and bloat, this fairly well proves that he should remain on the substitute milk. A number of babies will get better after a change to soy bean milk or goat's milk, but after a week or two start to scream and cry with cramps. Of course, they have become allergic to the new milk, and another substitute has to be tried.

(3) *Position.* Some babies do not like to be held when they are fed and seem to be irritated by any effort to soothe them. It is perfectly acceptable and *not* psychologically damaging to let your baby lie flat on his back or tipped slightly to the right with the bottle propped. Some mothers get quite skillful at thumping the baby's abdomen in the upper left portion—as if testing a melon. When the *thoonk* is just right, they know that he should be picked up and burped.

(4) *Nipple Holes.* Obviously nothing can be done about the nipple holes used by breast-fed babies, but many people assume that the manufacturers of bottle nipples calibrate them so that they are exactly the right size. This is not so. In general, they're too small. A way for you to test rubber nipples is to put cold formula in the bottle and turn the bottle upside down. Without shaking, the milk should drip out at the rate of about one drop a second. If this doesn't happen, the holes are too small and need enlarging. Using a knife, make a crosscut over the hole so that in essence there are four flaps in the nipple top. When your baby sucks, these flaps will open and let the milk flow to him quite rapidly. A baby swallows *more* air if the nipple holes are too small, because he sucks air *around* the nipple. If the holes are large or if the crosscut method is used, he'll get less air and less bloat. Breast-fed babies almost always get their milk at a rather rapid rate, so bottle milk should also come at a rapid rate to simulate Nature's way. The baby should be able to take almost all his quota in five to fifteen minutes.

(5) *Inadequate feeding.* I have had a few mothers who reported that their babies yelled with colic if they gave them what they thought was an adequate amount of milk (four to eight ounces). Because the bottles held only eight ounces, they assumed it was enough. But when offered ten ounces, the babies were completely satisfied. This seems like an outrageous amount for a small baby, but it is clearly what some babies

prefer. Before the mothers stumbled on this, they were offering six ounces five times a day, but the babies wanted ten ounces three times a day. They were perfectly happy when they finally received this amount. (Of course, their total twenty-four-hour intake was the same in each case.)

(6) *Obstructions.*   About one out of four babies is born with a slight narrowing of the anal-rectum junction, just one-half or one-fourth of an inch inside the anal opening. It acts as a partial obstruction. When the baby's stomach is filled with milk, a reflex begins bowel action in the colon. If there is even a slight obstruction to the passage of stool and gas through the anal opening, the baby usually doubles up and screams. He usually opens up this area after having passed a few stools, but sometimes you or the doctor have to pass a lubricated little finger inside his anus—probably no farther than an inch—to dilate the constricted area. If this is the cause of his distress, the baby will show immediate improvement. Sometimes this maneuver is accompanied by the passage of a drop or two of blood. Some mothers have found that their babies have pockets of gas inside the anal opening, and by passing in a glycerine suppository they can help the baby express the stool and gas. However, this only relieves some of the gas in the last six inches or foot of the colon, not in the twenty feet of intestine between the stomach and anus.

(7) *Nonintestinal causes.*   Because the urinary department is located in the abdomen, a congenital urinary obstruction can sometimes imitate colic. You should notify your doctor of any symptoms your child may have in this area—such as not being able to urinate for some hours at a time, or seeming to be in distress when he does urinate, or his urinary stream being thin and feeble. Any of these indicate some obstructive problem. The opening of the urethra at the head of the penis should be not just a pinhole but a slot usually

measuring about one-sixteenth of an inch. Sometimes a urine irritation or a urine burn can cause a stricture at the opening that results in back-pressure to the urinary stream, colic, and even damage to the kidneys. Be sure to inspect this opening to make certain that it is adequate.

When all efforts have failed to reduce the baby's screaming attacks and he seems to need to be carried around a great deal of the time, you should seek some medical relief. Most doctors will prescribe one of the barbiturates or a drug that has an effect on gastrointestinal spasms. These drugs seem to be quite safe if given in proper dosage, and can be given over some weeks or months without hurting your baby. He should outgrow his colic by the time he is three to six months old, but if he is really touchy, he may need some type of sedative medicine, tranquilizer, or antispasm medicine for some months or years after infancy.

I assume such overreactive babies simply notice their intestines more than others. I see babies who are burping, passing gas, and bloated, and it doesn't bother them at all. Others can get one little bubble in their intestinal tract and go wild: Their nervous systems are more easily stimulated.

Only after satisfactory milk feedings have been established should you begin to introduce solids. Years ago, babies were fed nothing but milk during their first year because there was nothing else convenient to give them. Milk was thought to be the perfect food, but since they were growing so fast these babies developed a terrible milk anemia because there is little, if any, iron in milk. Then companies began to make strained foods for babies, and parents began introducing them to their tots at an early age. Accordingly, babies no longer developed milk anemia, but a big race began to get them started on solids even earlier. This trend has now become so ridiculously exaggerated that it should be stopped. As Dr. J. B. Bilderback, the dean of pediatrics in Portland, Oregon, once told me, "Parents should at least wait until the cord is cut before they begin solids."

Although there are differences of opinion, most doctors feel that it's best not to be hasty about starting solid foods. One very

important reason for delay is related to food allergies—the earlier you start a food, the more likely it is that your baby will
develop an allergy to it. He may never be able to eat it for the
rest of his life, so in general, he'll be better off if he has no solids
to eat for the first few months. He gains faster on the milk, and
it provides the calcium and the calories he really needs during
this rapid growing phase. If a baby continued to grow at the same
rate he does during his first three weeks of life, by the age of ten
years he'd be twenty feet tall!

A number of the companies that prepare milk now add iron,
so it's even less important to start solid food early in life. If you
have a choice (i.e., if your child has no related milk allergies),
you should keep him on iron-enriched milk for the first six to
eight months of life.

If you *really* want to, it is permissible to start some solid food
around three or four weeks. Rice and barley are the safer ones.
They have a fair amount of calories, and they do help fill the
gaps. However, it will usually take you about twenty minutes to
get this cereal down your baby, and he'll probably sleep only
twenty minutes longer than he would have without it.

Many times I suggest to the mother of a five-week-old baby
that she start feeding him some solid foods, just to see if he will
sleep longer. "I've been giving him only milk," she will say, "and
last night he slept through the night for the first time in his life."
Babies are going to sleep through the night when they're good
and ready, which is when they stop growing so fast—it is as
simple as that. Adding a lot of solid food will not alter the sleep
pattern substantially, but it's all right to try a little cereal to see
if it helps.

Rice is somewhat more constipating, so if his stools are sloppy,
use rice. If his stools are rather firm, barley is probably a better
choice. Oatmeal is safe too, but many babies are very sensitive
to wheat, and this should be left out of his diet until he is much
older. I have found the safer fruits to be applesauce and bananas.
These are somewhat constipating, however, so if your baby's
stools are hard because of the milk he is drinking, it might be
better to try him on pears. However, although pears are usually
safe, the lemon juice added to them by the manufacturer often
causes upsets or rashes. Yellow vegetables are usually safe also.

Start only one new food a month, so that if any one causes trouble you will know which one it is. Another reason for waiting is that the extra solids put too much of a salt load on a baby's kidneys. Infant kidneys are immature and need plenty of water during the first few months of life to handle salts and minerals. If the amount of salt in his diet reaches a critical level in relation to the water, his kidneys will not be able to handle it. The salt is then stored, causing edema or dropsy. (This would only become a problem at times of sickness or hot, dry weather.)

In summary, it is best not to rush the starting of solids and to begin them slowly and cautiously. Again, the three reasons for caution are: (1) they do not do that much good, and your baby's physical equipment is designed mainly for milk, (2) it is likely that he may develop an allergy, and (3) some evidence indicates that solids provide too much salt for a baby's kidneys to handle.

Solid foods *should* be encouraged after your baby is six months of age, and milk should be discouraged at about the same time. Because of the previous problem I mentioned—the development of a milk anemia after six months of age—your best plan is to start the meal with solid foods and then give milk afterwards. An average six-month-old would perhaps take one or two jars of solid food a day divided into three feedings of breakfast, lunch, and dinner (a standard jar equals four ounces).

TYPICAL SIX-MONTH DIET

Breakfast	½ jar of fruit mixed with cereal
Lunch	½ jar of fruit
Dinner	½ jar of vegetables

The point is that your baby will decide how much milk he needs after eating the solids. I feel that milk is a bonus food at this age, and that the solids are more important.

There is some controversy about when to introduce meats in the diet. Many feel meat is worth starting early, because of its protein and iron content. But again, it may create quite a salt load, and your baby will be quite healthy even if he stays a vegetarian until his seventh or eighth month.

TYPICAL EIGHT-MONTH DIET

Breakfast	Four-ounce jar of fruit mixed with cereal, followed by two to eight ounces of milk
Lunch	Jar of mixed vegetables and beef or veal, followed by milk
Dinner	Jar of fruit or vegetables, possibly cereal and milk afterwards

After seven or eight months, a baby is usually on three jars of baby food a day; milk is given at the end of the meal. The amount of milk consumed is left up to him—if he cuts way down on his intake of milk, it's probably the best thing for him. The more milk he drinks after eight months of age, the more likely he is to develop a milk anemia. At ten months, your baby will often be on table food or be taking two jars of food three times a day.

TYPICAL TEN-MONTH DIET

Breakfast	Two jars of fruit, cereal, two to ten ounces of milk afterwards
Lunch	Two jars of mixed vegetables and beef, veal, or chicken with milk afterwards
Dinner	Two jars of fruit or vegetables, and milk afterwards

I have usually found that the foods I have mentioned are the safer ones. Do not give your baby citrus fruits or tomato juice. You should not give him peaches because they are likely to cause quite a rash either around the mouth and cheeks, or around the anal opening. Certainly, give no egg or wheat—they are both troublemakers. Green vegetables, peas, beans, and spinach should also be left alone until the baby is ten months to a year old. Many have found that their babies become allergic to those foods if they are given too soon, and the problem may never be outgrown. It is best to ignore them and start them later. No one food is ever vitally important or essential to the diet.

After six or eight months, babies can drink table milk, such as skim milk or milk containing 2 percent fat. The fat in the milk is the least important ingredient, and in the long run it is best not to have extra fat in the diet because of its known relationship to vascular disease. If your family can get used to drinking skim milk or milk with only 2 percent fat, your baby should drink this after eight to ten months.

Mothers of babies six or eight months old frequently ask, "Do you think he's getting enough fluid?" At about this time, the baby is beginning to cut down on his milk consumption. We know that in the first six to ten months of life, the baby's kidneys are not able to concentrate fluid very well. His urine is usually quite dilute, and he has to have a relatively large amount of fluid to carry off his wastes. This is supplied from the milk he drinks, which contains roughly 90 percent water. Up to six or eight months of age, if your baby is passing very dilute urine quite frequently, that's fine. Except in very hot parts of the country, extra water or juice is really not necessary. After eight or ten months, if he urinates at least three or four times a day, he's getting enough fluid. On very hot days, perhaps he should be given some extra—you can water down his milk or give extra juices.

You may well wonder about the ammonia smell that babies develop at this age. Because they sleep so well through the night, they really smell bad in the morning. Don't think, though, that if you give them extra fluids, the increased urine will wash away the smell. Actually, it will only make things worse: More urine allows the bacteria in the diaper to form more ammonia, and therefore more odor. The stronger the smell, the more burned your baby's bottom and the more blisters he will develop. Cutting down on his fluid usually will help this condition. (See ammoniacal diaper in the "Quick Reference Directory.")

Remember, milk is the main part of the diet during the first six or eight months, but less important afterwards. By the time your baby is a year old, milk is usually decreased considerably and can be considered a bonus food. If your baby is a good-size individual like you and your husband and eats an adequate amount of solid food (maybe close to six jars a day or the equivalent in table food), then it doesn't matter a great deal how much milk he takes. If he's small and is taking a fairly good amount of solids (three or more jars or their equivalent in table food, including some protein such as meat) then you can cut way down on his milk and offer little or none.

The most important part of the human diet is some kind of protein, such as meat, plus some fruits or vegetables. Animal protein is the best type and is better than that found in dairy products, nuts, or beans. Babies get iron, protein, and some vitamin B from meat, and some minerals and vitamin C from fruit. Of course, they need some extra vitamins during the period of rapid growth—the first eight or twelve months. There are not adequate vitamins in milk unless supplied artificially (the container will tell you), so you should give extra vitamins at this time. Fluoride is a problem in our country, and until we get it in all the water supplies it too must be supplied artificially and should be continued until at least eight years of age.

Once your fifteen- to eighteen-month-old baby is getting a reasonably adequate diet consisting mainly of meat and fruit or vegetables, he doesn't need vitamin supplements because there are enough in the food he eats. Again, the baby I worry about is the one who does nothing but drink milk, eat bread, and get anemic. The very foods that would correct the anemia become the ones he doesn't like. His mother says, "Well, milk is so good; so long as he drinks his milk, I don't care if he eats anything or not." This is the wrong approach. If he won't eat the other foods that are good for him and necessary for the prevention of anemia —such as meat and fruit or vegetables—then you should really make an effort to wean him from milk. In this way, he will be starved into eating the things that are better for him. But too many people take the easy way out, assuming that their child is healthy on a milk diet. He will not only become anemic, but almost always constipated as well.

Meal times should be enjoyable. If you make your child comfortable and let him understand that eating is a social affair, you are well on the way to inculcating good table manners and all that this entails. And, needless to say, the fewer hassles you have, the easier it will be to keep your baby contented and easy-going when he is away from the table.

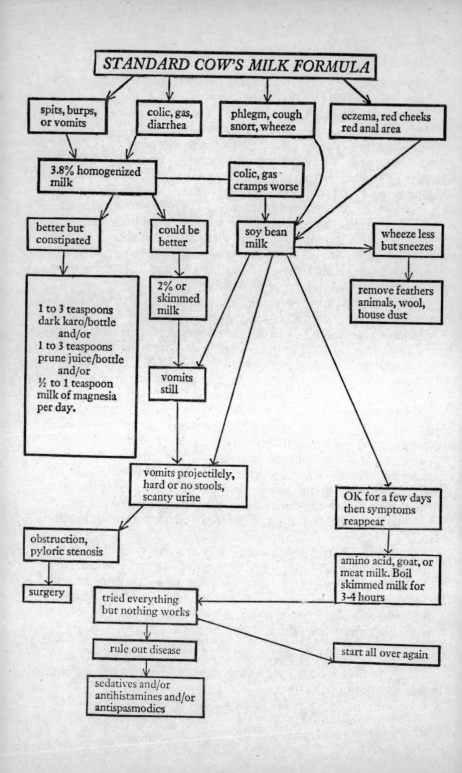

3 ◆◆◆◆

WHAT TO WATCH FOR
AND WHEN

"Or could it be he's going through a phase?"

Your children are intelligent, social animals. In order for your offspring to live with others *and* themselves, it is up to you to teach them human dignity, respect for life, and how to get their own way without hurting others. Parents, especially mothers, have to bring their children what little bits and pieces of education, religion, culture, and science they believe will help them achieve their potential with as little anxiety as possible.

The trick is to train your child to control his worst instincts—aggression, greed, and the like—without breaking his spirit. A growing child must be taught to control his impulses as soon as he begins to encroach on his environment.

The permissive school of child-rearing has lost ground because it tends to lead to impulse-ridden adults. I happen to believe you should set firm limits on your child's behavior; if you do not say "no" to him now, as an adult he will not be able to say "no" to himself. A mature adult has to postpone immediate gratification of his needs and drives—this is one of the main distinctions between us and the lower animals. It is also cheaper, and often keeps us out of jail.

Naturally, if you are aware of the various "phases" all children have to move through, you will be better equipped to guide your own child over the rocky road to adulthood. There is a phrase I keep coming back to that I hope you will remember, and maybe cut out and nail to the wall. This time-honored quote —whose origin is lost in antiquity—states simply that "Learning waits on maturation." Your child cannot learn something until his neuromuscular mechanism is mature enough to cope with that particular activity. For instance, a three-year-old is almost never able to cope with differential calculus—he is not mentally developed enough to handle the concepts. Too many of the things that we do at, for, and with our children seem to push them a little bit more than their capabilities can handle.

When your child doesn't measure up to some level or standard that you think he's ready for, you will find that standard is often based on what your neighbor's child can do. This attitude is often as frustrating for your child as it is for you.

As a particular example, a mother may rush over to her neighbor's house with the glad news that her child has been toilet-trained at eighteen months! (She has just caught a couple of stools in the potty.) Of course the neighbor, whose two-and-a-half-year-old stubbornly refuses to go near the toilet, is miffed and discouraged. She now feels inferior in her child-rearing efforts, and so gets more aggressive in trying to toilet-train her own child—which naturally makes him rebel all the more. The house is plunged into hostility and turmoil by her attempt to keep up with the toilet-trained Joneses.

What *doesn't* happen two weeks later is significant. That neighborhood mother *should* come back and painfully admit that her eighteen-month-old is not toilet-trained after all—as is almost always the case. The mother may have caught a stool or two, but then her child learned he was doing something his mother wanted him to do, so he quit. Of course she won't really have him trained until he is two and a half or three years of age. But she is not going to let her neighbor know that her child failed her, especially after she has gone around and said that he *was* trained. This would certainly be a loss of face, a loss of status. At least the mother of the untrained child had not claimed success.

You must somehow accept your child as an individual and not

WHAT TO WATCH FOR AND WHEN   35

show disappointment when he seems to compare unfavorably with siblings or neighboring children. The wise mother allows her child to grow at his own pace. Remember that it takes about twenty years to climb to maturity, and each step is built on the successful completion of the previous one.

Research indicates that a healthier personality develops if *positive* rewards are given for success. Your love and enthusiasm reinforces your growing infant who says "mama" or who takes his first step. It develops his self-esteem better than if you carped constantly at his soiling, messing, thumb-sucking, or tantrums. This same positive concentration on the good in your growing child is valuable all through his life. If his leisurely attainments meet with constant disappointment, he will only learn to devalue himself—"I must be really wicked for Mamma to make such a fuss." Such a child will never be successful in his own mind, and will become a nit-picker or a moody defeatist, or even develop bodily symptoms.

Neuromuscular maturity proceeds from top to bottom. Your newborn baby is provided with only the essential life-saving reflexes and functions—heartbeat, respiration, sucking, swallowing, hunger cry, and withdrawal response to pain. His neck and head control appear first. Purposeful arm movements and grasping are next. When the lower back muscles are responsive to the brain's messages, your baby can sit (six to nine months). His legs are next on the list, but walking will not be accomplished until the nervous system has matured enough to tell the leg muscles what to do.

Only after the toddler toddles can you expect him to handle his bladder and bowel functions with the same finesse. Toilet training only achieves neatness—it is sort of a luxury item, on a pretty low priority next to walking and verbal communication.

This, of course, is why parents are usually frustrated when they attempt it too early. A child has to have neuromuscular control first, then he has to see how it is done, then he has to *want* to do it because you (who love him) want him to do so.

As the muscles become hooked up with the brain and functioning, the child comes to grips with his environment. With your guidance he will learn that the world can be dangerous. Stoves may be hot. Streets can have cars that barrel along. Knives often cut skin. Gravity always works. A mother is like the doe who has to teach her fawn about the nasty, carnivorous puma. Your child has to test his environment to learn which things hurt and which give pleasure. He will learn to control his anger and hostility because you disapprove. He must channel these feelings into socially acceptable pursuits that are rewarded by approval and love. The maturing child has to be exposed to them so he can receive feedback. By the time he is six years old, his adaptive responses are quite well formed; his personality has developed. After this, he attempts various refinements and minor readjustments—some successfully, others not. He learns most of the rules by breaking them. You should therefore be nearby to referee this game your child is playing—it is called "experience."

You will constantly look for reassurance that your child is bright—not just average, but bright. You can tell your friends you don't care as long as he is *average*, but way down deep you really hope he is bright, that he's sharp, that he'll make it in this world and show off his great parental care and genetic background. Obviously, you're the ones who made this all possible. So, I would like to give you some guidelines, things that you can watch for, as indications that your child is at least of average intelligence. I may not be able to reassure you that he is brighter than average. You can draw that conclusion yourself, if you can risk being disappointed later on to find he is just a normal, average adult.

ONE MONTH

At one month of age, a baby is still pretty much a sucking reflex with a loud mouth at one end and no responsibility at the other. His head often still sags. An object put in his hand will drop out. He stares indefinitely into space. If you are worried because you think he may have vision trouble, wait a while. If you are holding the baby out at arm's length and he's looking over your shoulder, don't assume that he is ignoring you or that he is blind. If you are less than a yard away, you are simply a blurry blob to him since he cannot focus. Usually after six weeks to two months, babies have a social smile and can distinguish a face from a football. Then test his eyes with a bright light. If he flinches, assume his gross vision is normal. He will make some responses to loud, sharp noises. If he does not do so even after one month of age, it may not mean anything, but you should be suspicious of hearing trouble.

Apparently, the two most important things you are supposed to do for a baby at this age are to feed and love him. You are supposed to get a little bit tired, and it's normal to complain about the hard work he necessitates. But he is just sweet and dependent enough that he brings out the mother in you, and you can forgive him for waking you up at night and creating a lot of laundry. If you are at all normal, you cannot help but love this little warm lump of humanity. (If a mother cannot love her baby, they are both in serious trouble.) He does just enough cute things to make you want to show him off. This foundation of love and respect has to be established in these first few months, because everything the mother and child will do for each other is based on this early "affair."

TWO MONTHS

At two months of age a baby is almost surely able to look at his hands or fix his gaze on some moving object near his eyes. He may even be able to open his hands and take hold of objects, but he will usually drop them. His head does not sag forward when he is propped up; however, it may jerk around. He is usually still sleeping and eating a lot, but also having some wakeful moments when he is not screaming from hunger. He seems to enjoy having company and is beginning to become a pleasure to have around. This is a very important time, and psychologists tell us you should stimulate and play with him by tickling him and singing, talking, and making some contact. How can you help responding and being overjoyed by the mere fact of being the mother of a small baby who is completely dependent? Most women need to be needed and love to be loved, and a two- to six-month-old baby fulfills your great drive more than anything else in the whole world. Make the most of it! Love has a lot to do with the child's security later on in life, and a great deal to do with his intellectual and communicative abilities.

This seems to be a quite well-documented fact. If a mother stimulates her child, talks and sings to him, even though she uses nonsense words and cannot sing on key, the child benefits. His brain needs to have messages going through it from the many different sensory pathways to his nervous system. The opposite is quite true. If no one stimulates a baby and he is left all alone in his bed, he may not attain his full mental potential even though he receives adequate physical care. Even television and radio provide some stimulation.

THREE MONTHS

Three months of age is the delightful age of infancy, especially for the pediatrician. These children laugh and smile at everybody, even doctors. I am amazed at how a baby laughs and smiles at other, older children more than he does at the mother who is feeding him, changing him, and making him comfortable. He really seems to enjoy their attention more, even when these older children are real roughnecks. They will poke and pinch and drag an infant around the floor, but the baby will love it and laugh heartily. Unless he really gets hurt, he thinks it's great fun. Children know how to communicate with one another. Sometimes they don't seem to get along very well, but I have a feeling they realize they're all together in this battle against adults. They're always happy to discover another recruit. The infant senses this and feels he's somehow on their side.

At this age, the baby's eyes will follow objects. He laughs and gets excited at different stimuli, and has a very definite social smile. He has discovered his hands and finds them fascinating. His head is pretty steady when he is on his stomach, and he can lift it up at a ninety-degree angle to look around. He can get stimulated by the sight of a toy and even grab it and stick it in his mouth. These things usually happen by the time a child is four months old, so between three and six months is the best time for taking pictures of him or taking him to visit in-laws. This is better than waiting until he is over eight months. At the earlier age the baby thinks that just about anything that is human is pretty terrific. Your baby cries more in the presence of the *paternal* grandmother, so if you are having a little trouble relating to your mother-in-law, you might try letting her see him when he is between three and five months of age. She can be the ugliest old crab in the world, but the baby will smile and laugh at her. If you are traveling or moving, your baby can tolerate it better at this age than when he is a little older. Usually he is sleeping through the night by this time, and intestinal problems are pretty well straightened out. If you have worked out a schedule of naps and play, he is usually well-settled into a routine.

FOUR TO FIVE MONTHS

By the time your baby is in his fourth month, his individual personality is quite obvious to everyone. He can be relied upon to have certain responses in certain situations, and he usually has a good laugh when he sees you. He likes to focus his eyes and grab colored moving objects. He gets excited when he thinks you are going to play games with him.

I remember reading in a book on child psychology published rather recently that a baby should *never* be tickled. The author's view was that a baby should laugh and be happy only because of a deep-down sense of security. He thought that laughter in response to a pleasant skin stimulation was artificial, superficial, and very bad indeed. Well, mothers enjoy patting their baby dry after his bath, playing peek-a-boo with him, and maybe giving him a kiss on the back of the neck. The baby gets to laughing because he is tickled, and mother and baby have a great time giggling with each other. An insecure mother reading the above article might feel that she had been doing something wrong to the child's psyche. Hopefully, few mothers have seen the article and baby tickling will continue to flourish.

If you are intuitive, you will know your child's personality well enough by this age to be able to sense whether he is sick or well, happy or unhappy. You will be aware of behavior and activity changes that you may not be able to define verbally except to say, "He's different; something is wrong." Your doctor must find the reason and correct it when you say so, because you are usually right.

Somewhere around the fourth or fifth month, a baby starts to drool and slobber. It is thought that this is a sign he's about to cut some teeth, but as far as I can tell, this drooling and slobbering is just the result of increased saliva flow at about this age. Since saliva does not taste that good, and since he is not too concerned about being socially acceptable, he just lets it run out of his mouth. He also notices that somebody keeps mopping it up, so it becomes a good way to get attention. The teeth themselves almost always come after six months.

Around this time, a child likes to be propped up with pillows or put in a baby seat so he can have a view of what's going on around him. He cannot sit by himself yet and often leans forward on his stomach or tips over on his side as if he had a round bottom. This is when one of the most famous old wives' tales disturbs the new mothers who intuitively feel it is perfectly all right to prop the baby. Grandmother often comes over to say that if you prop up a baby, he'll get hunch-backed because he doesn't have enough calcium in his spine. This is a lot of nonsense. If your baby is not screaming when he is propped up, then his back muscles and his backbone are perfectly all right, even if he does look sloppy. Of course he slouches, but it doesn't hurt him. If he is happy observing the environment, he should be encouraged and propped—it's another way to provide stimuli to his nervous system.

A baby in a playpen should have some stimulating toys. You should be nearby to talk to the child occasionally, and his playpen should not be used as a form of solitary confinement. In countries where mothers take washing down to the stream or stand in line for shopping, they take their babies along in a sling on their backs. It certainly provides a great chance for mother and child to talk or laugh. Anything goes, just as long as they keep the lines of communication open. Stimulation is so important at this age (and the age passes so quickly) that I probably should reemphasize it. *Sensory communication is vital, whether it be auditory, visual, or tactile.*

SEVEN MONTHS

At seven months of age, a normal baby is able to sit, leaning forward on his outstretched arms. When held in the standing position, he will bounce up and down, bending his knees. He is usually able to grasp toys at this age and will take a rattle with one hand instead of using the two-handed method he used earlier. When crying, he usually makes a "mm-mmm" noise, and there may be a few vowel sounds. If a mirror is placed in front of him, he will often reach out and try to be sociable with his image.

At just about seven or eight months of age, a very distressing thing seems to happen. The baby starts to develop a temper, a little stubbornness to his personality. He seems to say, "Well, things aren't going my way and I think I'll fight for my rights a little bit." If you take a toy away, he often responds rather vocally. Equally disturbing at seven to nine months of age is his reaction when you leave him alone to take his nap or to go to sleep for the night.

To me, this is a more important indication of a child's development than his learning to sit or stand. A child at this age suddently realizes that he is not attached to his mother by some magical umbilical cord. When he's left alone, he thinks that you're gone forever and he really gets scared. His response is a heart-breaking wail. You may rush in, thinking he has hurt himself, but naturally he is all smiles when you lift him up.

A wise mother says, "Ah! So this is the kind of deal you're working! Well, I'm sorry, but it's bedtime and you are going to go down and go to sleep. I'll see you later when it's time to get up." So she puts him down again, and sure enough he screams. At this age the baby is *supposed* to do this, if he is normal. And his mother, being wiser than the child, should know that she must leave him there; he must work out this problem for himself.

How well you and your child get through this irritating phase depends on his personality and your confidence and endurance. You will have difficulty getting out of the house because the child raises such a commotion. At this point, it is probably best if he sees as few strangers as possible, since he is so easily upset by them. Again, this is part of the normal maturing process—it is probably a good sign that his intelligence is close to normal.

NINE TO TEN MONTHS

People think a baby should sit at six months and walk at twelve months, but this is not universally so. I was trained to ask the mother, "When was your baby able to sit so well that you could leave the room and come back and find him still sitting?" That is nine and a half months. Some babies, of course, sit well at five months and can even walk at seven months. One mother told me that her child was *walking* at seven months. His feet were far apart, but he walked well and was quite stable. To see this tiny child hiking around the room was really a sight.

At the time, I assumed that children who walked early would grow up to be well-coordinated adults or even acrobats. So I asked the mother, "Is this a hereditary thing? Were you able to walk early?"

"Yes," she said, "I was an early walker. I walked well by the time I was six months old."

"Aha!" I said, "What are you now? A famous acrobat?"

"No," she replied, "I'm quite clumsy. I can't even open a can without getting cut."

Thus, early maturation indicates that intelligence is normal or average, but is no special indication of superiority. Many prodigies have burned themselves out later. Of course, it is more difficult to generalize about a child who *doesn't* sit well until he is ten months old, doesn't stand until the sixteenth month, and doesn't take a step until the twentieth. He is more likely to be at least mildly retarded than the child who follows the norm. In general, though, muscular coordination is not the only index of future abilities. We make so many mistakes in trying to determine a young child's intelligence that most of us avoid predictions. Usually we can reassure a mother that her child is *probably* within normal limits. A child's social awareness at ten months (screaming when isolated, upset when faced with a stranger) may be a better clue of intelligence than the age at which he sits, stands, and walks. Physical, mental, and social growth, adaptive abilities, and environment must all be considered when making an assessment—and even then you can be wrong.

A ten-month-old is quite good at creeping, and many are able to pull themselves to their feet. Their verbalizations usually are fairly clear-cut, especially "mama," and "dada." They seem to say these words with meaning if their hearing is at all normal. Usually they are able to wave bye-bye and can sometimes even "patty cake" on request. Most female babies are starting to feed themselves by this time, since girls are usually a little faster in their development and manipulative ability than boys. Up to age two, the girl is usually one month ahead.

When your baby begins to crawl, you must carefully check his environment for all possible hazards that have become available to him through his new mobility. You should remove from his reach all sorts of poisons, bottles, machinery, and anything else that might be dangerous. I am especially concerned about the mother who loads up the coffee table with a lot of bric-a-brac and things that she does not want her child to touch. Of course, they are such a great attraction that he is right there eating cigarette butts and smashing things to the floor. The mother whales into him with a lot of "no's" and smacks him right and left. I think this is a dirty trick—the mother should have kept these things out of his way in the first place.

One good system is to get down on your hands and knees, even if this seems rather silly, and look at the world from your child's viewpoint. All those lovely soaps and poisons and bleaches that you keep under the kitchen sink are right at his eye level, and are, of course, attractive. It is "monkey see, monkey do." If he sees you using the soap and bleach, then he will want to do it, too, because he thinks that you are having a lot of fun and it will be fun for him, too (except he will want to drink them). Crawl around and look in all the corners for poisons and various sharp objects with which your child could hurt himself. In this technological age, we have hot hair dryers, explosive aerosol cans, and mercury vapor tubes ("fluorescent lights") that implode in a cloud of poisonous powder. These items do not seem hazardous to us simply because we read and heed the label. Remember, though, that it took much needless grief to convince the public what a plastic bag can do. Use your imagination. If it is not safe to eat, take apart, pull over your head, or slam around, it will not be good for your baby, so get it out of the way.

Another thing worth thinking about is what to do in an emergency. You should make a dry run: Find out how close you are to the fire department (where they have oxygen), the hospital (where they could treat bleeding, burns, or respiratory trouble), and the doctor's office. At least be able to contact a doctor by phone. You should work out such arrangements in advance. If you are really out in the country, you must make some sort of plan for transportation. Either develop some arrangement with a neighbor or make sure a car is available should you need fast help.

ONE YEAR

By the time they are one year old, almost all children insist on feeding themselves. Here is another behavior principle we know: A child will do something not only when he is mature enough to do it, but when he sees someone else doing it.

I had two children as patients who were fed in their room by their nurse. Their nurse did not eat with them, so they never had an opportunity to see an adult feeding himself. I guess they assumed that everybody in the world got fed by someone else. When they were about three or four, their mother decided to send them to nursery school. All went well until the midmorning snack. When served their juice and cookies, they just sat there passively because they expected somebody to feed it to them. Looking around the room, they saw the other children gobbling down the cookies and drinking the juice. "Oh," they realized, "*that's* the way it's done. You use your hands to put it in your mouth!" And so they did.

This was fantastic to me, since I thought that if you are hungry it is a natural instinct to grab food, put it in your mouth, and swallow it. Perhaps this was an isolated example. Still, I sometimes wonder whether children would ever learn to stand up if their elders crawled around on all fours.

In any case, feeding a one-year-old is rather distressful if you are a neat, compulsive mother. I know it would be a lot easier, quicker, and neater for you to shovel the food in with a spoon, but your child has to learn to do it. He will grab the spoon or get his fingers in the sloppy baby food. In very short order, there will be a sticky mess all over the room. Also, he will test gravity over and over again. The one-year-old's eating behavior must be derived from some sort of genetic memory of the early cave dwellers who might have grabbed a mouse, squeezed it, and smashed it against the floor of the cave. Then, if it did not move, it could be eaten. The modern child does this with a banana or boiled carrot: grab, squeeze, smash. Then, if it looks dead lying on the table or squishes out invitingly between the fingers, it can be eaten. Of course, you don't have to worry that he'll never use knife, fork, and spoon; if you use a knife, fork, and spoon, your child will eventually do the same. He has to go through the messy feeding stage when he is about a year old. Rest assured: When he is mature enough to use the spoon, he will. Most mothers learn to feed their year-old children lumpy foods, things they can pick up in their hands. So, breakfast can be a hunk of banana or some applesauce and dry cereal stuck together. Lunch might be a peanut-butter-and-jelly sandwich, and supper could be some ground meat, a few French-fried potato sticks, a few peas, a slice or two of boiled carrot.

Punishing a child of this age for messing with his food only serves to make mealtime unhappy when its chief benefit, next to nourishment, should be the joy of companionship and communication. Serving small portions of finger foods in a saucer should help prevent some of the mess. If he is still hungry, he will indicate this to you. Let him ask you for more. Don't urge him to eat. Don't punish him for the spill that *you* allowed—his neuromuscular control has not developed sufficiently. He does not seem to understand that by the time he has filled his spoon and swung it up to where his mouth is supposed to be, the spoon is upside down and empty. Showing wrath for his inability to succeed will make him feel as you did on the first day on the job when the boss said, "Turn the toggle switch on the cam device."

FIFTEEN MONTHS

An average child takes his first step at fifteen months. That may seem rather late to most people, but it turns out to be average. Many perfectly normal children are not able to take a step until they are eighteen months old. We get a little nervous if they have not taken a step after that age, but it is still compatible with being normal.

With his first step, your child immediately becomes a toddler. He observes, hears, tastes, and feels his environment. He has to learn what is safe and what is dangerous in the world. You cannot tell him; he has to experience it so it becomes part of him but your presence is necessary so the experiments will not be fatal.

There is a strange feeling that comes over most parents, that once a child starts to walk, he is out of babyhood. They feel that he should be able to act a little more like an adult, understand what "no" means, and respect the property rights of others. But a child of this age has virtually no conception of these things, and his mother finds that all she is saying to him is, "No!"

You *should* say "no" to a child whenever he oversteps the bounds of reasonable social living. "No" should be used vigorously and repeatedly—and emphasized with some physical punishment if necessary—but only when necessary. Make an effort to provide an environment for your child in which "no" is used as little as possible. Some day when he is about to step into the path of a truck, you will say "no" and want him to freeze. But he won't do so if you have used the word excessively and without meaning.

Don't view him as an adult. He cannot control his own impulses at this age. Make "no" something important, but give him a few "yes's," too. I think its important for him to have someplace in the house (maybe in his room and away from your best china) where he can do anything he wants and nobody will say "no" to him. I feel everybody needs a place they can go for a good cry, to be alone, or to sit quietly and meditate about life and its frustrations.

By fifteen months, a child is supposed to be able to creep up a step. He is supposed to be able to put one cube on top of another. He may have two to four words in his vocabulary, but his speech is generally an unintelligible word salad. But the most characteristic thing about a fifteen-month-old is his wild temper tantrums. He loves to investigate the obvious "no-no's." You may try to save him from danger, but he won't appreciate your efforts. When hauled away from the hot stove because "no!" didn't work, he has a temper tantrum. He stiffens out on the floor, kicks his heels, and wails as if stabbed.

The reasonable mother knows that it is just a fit of temper, that he is supposed to have these tantrums. It is his way of communicating hostility toward restrictions imposed on him. Almost everything he has done from birth has been an attempt to communicate with his environment—mainly the humans in it, and his mother especially. Everything he sees, feels, or hears evokes some response, and he reacts instinctively at the particular level of maturity available to his nervous system. But because his speech is limited, he has to throw a fit to indicate his frustrations. I feel that if he knew how to swear, he would not cry so much. To minimize his unforeseen difficulties, his environment and discipline should be as consistent as possible. If you disciplined your child one way on Monday, you should punish him in the same way when he commits the same "crime" on Wednesday. He feels more secure if he knows what the limits are, even though they may be restrictive. Children seem to ask for limits even though they continue to test them—witness the toddler who knows of the dangers of fire, gets near the oven, puts his hand cautiously out, looks at his mother, and says, "No, no."

While you are trying to civilize this animal, you sometimes get a little frantic knowing there is a deadline. The frustrating part is that once he has been properly disciplined for being "off limits" and has seemed to get the idea that, "If you do that again, I'll spank you," he does it again! He doesn't seem to learn. But, of course he has. What he's doing is testing, just making sure. Be patient and persistent and consistent; don't forget that a new phase will come along to replace this "testing" one, but it will undoubtedly be just as aggravating.

EIGHTEEN MONTHS

Once your child sees that temper tantrums are not rewarding —at about eighteen months—he stops this exhausting procedure. Then *he* begins to use the word "no," the one he has heard so frequently. His neuromuscular skills are growing, and he soon channels his energy into capitalizing on them. The girl talks more and begins to use language effectively to get what she wants. The boy is more active—climbing, running, jumping— and more physically aggressive. He can run a little clumsily and maybe even climb stairs if he holds on. He can now use a spoon and drink from a cup. He can recognize a few objects in pictures and a few parts of his body. A boy should have five words, a girl at least ten.

TWO YEARS

Almost on the exact day he turns two, the child begins to whine. It's almost as if he had read the book, his timing is so good. He soon discovers this form of communication gets a bigger rise out of you than what he was doing before. It is a new game he has discovered—he acts, you always react. He knows, for instance, that you would like him to stop sucking his thumb. He may even want to quit, and will be playing happily with his toys when you come into view. Immediately he pops the thumb into his mouth and starts to whine. It is like electronic feedback —the reaction occurs as soon as you see each other. The final straw is your mother-in-law, who says, "He never whines or sucks his thumb when *I* have him." The situation is usually aggravated at two years because you would like to initiate toilet training (another pressure to conform). Also at about this time, a child's appetite decreases so that he eats only about one-third as much as he had been eating a few months before—another frustrating event for Mother. Somehow, you will have to stop the cycle, interrupt the feedback.

Fortunately, verbal communication is now becoming more effective on both sides. Your child can vent his hostilities and gripes without so many direct explosions. He talks to his toys and develops his own play and drama therapy. The "acting out" also ventilates his psyche—it is healthy and should be encouraged. By the age of two years, he should be able to run and climb well. His span of attention is usually long enough for him to use scissors, draw a line, and listen to a short story. He insists on things going his way or else it is, "I no want." He is in serious trouble, possibly with hearing, if he does not have a good number of clearly pronounced words that he uses properly.

Psychologists and educators have indicated that much can be done for and with the infant and toddler's brain. Five to fifteen points can be added to a child's IQ score if early stimulation is effected. Because these enthusiastic researchers cannot get into your home, you are supposed to do the job yourself. Not every mother can; as a matter of fact, most find that they dissolve in tears along with their child if they try to be a teacher at home. Further problems can develop when a mother who has ineptly pushed her child's education enrolls him in the first grade. Either he is way ahead and thus bored, or he has forgotten it all and is just like any other normal six-year-old child.

The problem children who really need early stimulation live in homes where there is little intellectual excitement in the first place—few books, less reading, no art, poor music. In these depressing, deprived, disadvantaged homes, the conversation—what there is of it—is monosyllabic. Somebody has to sneak into such culturally barren homes and stimulate the infants and toddlers. It is too late to try with five- or six-year-olds; they will be behind for the rest of their lives. As adults, they feel cheated somehow because they cannot compete for "good" jobs. They blame their education for not getting them there. And in turn, they are unable to stimulate their children creatively because they are not too stimulating themselves. The problem is self-perpetuating.

Conversely, mothers who are well-read enough to be aware of

the advantages of early "creative play" are *already* stimulating their children, because it would not occur to them to behave otherwise. These mothers do things with their children in a happy "game-playing" way that is appropriate to the age. They urge without pushing. Their children are education-oriented and comfortable when the time comes for nursery school and kindergarten.

Remember, learning waits on maturation, and frustration follows failure due to neuromuscular inability. If you are "in tune" with your child, you will know how far to go, how much you can push. Motivation by rewards and love is strong in early childhood and is a happy introduction to nursery school and kindergarten—where competition for love and praise from the "teacher-mother" is the compelling learning force.

THREE YEARS

By age three, the exhausted mother is yearning to enroll her child in nursery school. She claims she wants to get him "ready for school and learn to relate to his peers," but at least 50 percent of her motivation is to get him out of the house. She loves him but cannot always like him. If you can admit this latter feeling, I think you are normal—and honest. I worry when a mother says she has *never* become angry with her child; I must assume she is covering up for a really deep hostility. Also, if she is constantly worrying that her child is afflicted with a fatal disease (which he is not), it may frequently suggest a neurotic attitude, a sick kind of wishful thinking.

In any case, it is important that your child get to nursery school. The new experiences he receives from a skilled teacher and other children put him way ahead when first grade comes around. Nursery school is frequently a good way to undeprive the disadvantaged child. A teacher can spot physical, neurological, and psychological difficulties to which a mother may be blind, at a time when remedies may be more rapidly effective.

Frequently, the child arrives home full of happy successes and announces, "Teacher says we should say, 'Thank you,'" or "Teacher says we should have good manners." The mother without a sense of humor can only cry when she hears this; she thought *she* has been teaching her child the rules of living, too.

A child of this age is eager to learn, but seems to tune out the mother. Direct orders have to be shouted or bells have to be rung to get attention. Sometimes this twist works—but only once: if you want him to go out, try, "Do you want to go out the front door or the back door?"

The nursery school teacher often judges the three-year-old's ability to ride a tricycle as a clue to his muscular coordination. If he cannot ride successfully, he may have a faulty nervous system. If he does not enjoy group play, he may be different, but might also have some abnormal personality trait. He can usually draw a circle or a spiral; he can undress himself. In the doctor's office, he is friendly and cooperative during the examination. If we are not too rough and he is not too anxious, the experience is a happy one and sets the tone for future pleasant doctor-patient relationships.

FOUR YEARS

The four-year-old likes to test the magic of words. He has heard his mother say to his father, "Shut the door," or "Come and eat," and as if by magic, these things happen. So *he* tries to communicate with the world and soon learns what works and what does not. "Shut!" he says to the door; it doesn't. "Drop dead!" he says to his mother; hopefully she doesn't. (If, for some reason, she *does* die soon after his command, he feels guilty forever. My most reasonable advice is to stay alive.) Again, he is testing his environment in a safe way so as to be more secure in his home. If you misinterpret these attempts at verbal control, you will not help your child pass this stage successfully. A wise mother accepts these sometimes irritating mouthings as nothing more than verbal horseplay and allows them to be rightfully forgotten.

Soon another method of exchange takes place, from "what?" to "why?" I can remember when one of my boys asked "Why?". Trying to be a nice father, I launched into a rather involved explanation. He interrupted with impatience and said, " 'Cuz." He was playing the communication game; he had said, "Why?" and I was supposed to answer, "Because." This was just the right answer for his age. (Our questions and answers have since become more involved; but you have to start someplace.)

Usually the four-year-old has become skilled enough to be a bit of a show-off, at least when around a three-year-old. He can draw a head and a couple of parts and call it a "man." A boy is quite proud of his ability to urinate in the toilet. (About 20 percent is on the floor, but he's too busy to worry about that.) He can tell a story and particularly likes scary ones—if they are not *too* frightening. They are a way to experience vicarious danger.

FIVE TO SIX YEARS

The five- to-six-year-old really needs to test property rights and the mine/not mine concept. Because stealing is a crime in our capitalistic society, you had better teach him respect for others' property and the concept of earning what he wants to possess. A child *takes* what he wants: *Stealing* sounds a little too grown up. He must sense that he is doing something wrong because he leaves enough clues about so that his "crime" will be discovered. It is a game similar to the one Dostoevski describes in *Crime and Punishment*—do something wrong; let somebody find out; get caught; feel guilty; get punished; have your guilt assuaged.

A confident mother who has insight into her child's phases will be able to endure them with some humor. She will be smart enough to disregard suggestions, comparisons, and criticisms from in-laws, neighbors, and friends. Every mother-child relationship is unique and defies comparison; what may be perfectly appropriate in one home is ridiculously absurd in another. If you provide love and limits and correlate learning with maturation, your home will nurture the child's personality. An attitude of casual concern, studied nonchalance, calculated indifference, subtle firmness, sneaky control, and bull-headed softness will pay off.

I assume you want your child to be a cautious rebel—to get happiness out of life's adventure, experience what the world has to offer without too much anxiety, enjoy his full potential without hurting anyone, and win more than he loses. Play the game properly, and you will find you have won, if you lose your son or daughter in marriage to someone with a few of your own good qualities.

DEVELOPMENTAL MAP

Age	Tests & Immunizations	Diet	Motor Development
1 MONTH	D.P.T. (1)	Milk, 2 ounces per pound per 24 hours Vitamins, fluoride, and Iron.	Cries, sucks, swallows, blinks at lights. Head sags, clenches hands.
2 MONTHS	Oral Polio D.P.T. (2)	Rice or Barley	Stares at objects, follows object with eyes.
3 MONTHS	Oral Polio D.P.T. (3)	Applesauce	Listens to sounds, raises head when prone "Social smile," smiles and laughs at people
3-5 MONTHS		Bananas Carrots	Rolls over Looks at and reaches for toy Follows object 180° Laughs and squeals
6-7 MONTHS		Squash Give solid foods first	Sits, leaning on hand Transfers cube from hand to hand Turns when spoken to or when someone speaks
8-9 MONTHS		Sweet potato Veal, beef, or lamb Teething biscuit	Sits well Stands, hanging on Thumb-finger grasp Imitates speech Shy with strangers Resists toy removal Plays peek-a-boo Cries upon separation
ONE YEAR to 15 MONTHS (FEMALE) — 28-30 inches at 1 year (MALE) — 29-31 inches at 1 year	Hemoglobin test Measles vaccine Smallpox vaccination Urine test	"Finger food" Discourage milk Cup Messes in food Egg, citrus, green vegetables, peaches	Feeds self; creeps Shows temper Pull up to sitting Cries on separation Waves "bye-bye"; imitates gestures Stands with support Crawls well; says "mama", "bye-bye" Walks alone; investigates

What Environment Should Provide	Warning, Suggestions, Comments
Touch, skin contact, motion, rocking Sounds to hear—especially human voices Objects to see—especially mother Full stomach, social contact Love, warmth, cuddling, security	Try to breast-feed Take a nap when he does Don't push solids—they're not important yet Baby should gain one to three pounds over birthweight
Sucking pleasure (pacifier or thumb) Mobiles, TV, pictures, things to see Voices, songs, records, simple stories Smiles and laughter when he smiles Human voices to talk when he talks People to watch Toys to excite him	Carry him about house and to store and park Do simple vision and hearing tests Good age to travel Good age to photograph him Don't leave him where he may fall
Pillow to prop him up to see and grasp Toys to grab Sling or chair so his feet touch the floor Handy objects to fondle and bite Human contact	Toys too big to swallow (remove buttons) No lead in paint He develops a temper Get used to separation cry
Needs mother or some baby sitter Reward and praise for accomplishment	Don't force spoon Don't wean suddenly Keep from undue contact with strangers

DEVELOPMENTAL MAP (Continued)

Age	Tests & Immunization	Diet	Motor Development
18 MONTHS to 2 YEARS (Double body length to estimate adult height; do this at 18 months for girls and 2 years for boys)	TB test D.P.T. Booster	Spoon Milk and white foods are *least* important Appetite decreases Meats, fruits, and fluoride *most* important One meal a day	Climbs stairs one at a time; kicks ball Says "no," pulls toy Three to five words Scribbles; uses cup without spilling Names objects in picture Bladder and bowel control Runs Sentences of three words Builds tower of several blocks Knows name Turns pages, uses scissors, can draw a line
3 YEARS	TB test Dentist	Definite food likes and dislikes	Draws circle, cross Rides tricycle, asks "what"
4 to 5 YEARS	Hearing test	Appetite better Serve small amounts; let him ask you for seconds	Can draw a man Plays with peers; can count three objects Balances on one foot for ten seconds Can jump on one foot, catch ball Prefers to play with other children Can tell a story
5 YEARS (Grows 2-3 inches a year)	Visual Acuity Test Oral Polio D.P.T. Booster Mumps Vaccine TB Test	3 reasonably good meals a day Meats most important; then fruits; then vegetables; then grain and cereal Milk and white foods least important	Imitates adult activity Asks "why" Interest in sex differences Throws ball Knows three or four colors Dresses and undresses self Copies some letters Can tell a longer story

What Environment Should Provide	Warning, Suggestions Comments
Consistent "no" or punishment for doing dangerous things	Read to him Start using toothbrush
Safe place to play, use muscles, and run—and have temper tantrums	He needs to mess in and smash food, imitate housework
Chance to scribble and smear without adult supervision	Remove poisons, paints, detergents, medicines (have syrup of Ipecac ready)
Answers to questions; ask him to name objects	Ignore temper tantrums
Nighttime rituals: tooth brushing, relaxing bath, story, cuddly animal, favorite blanket, prayers	Turn pot handles around on stove
	Bad time to stop pacifier or thumb sucking—he's too stubborn
Love and limits	
Honest answers about sex and parts of body	Girl may be toilet-trainable
Reassurance or night light to counter sleep resistance, fear of the dark	If he won't eat and suffers constipation, stop milk and white foods
	Whining begins, try to ignore it

Nursery school or constructive social play	Stammering common; pretend you don't notice
Increased periods of separation from parents	Rely on your sense of humor when he calls you names
Praise for verbal accomplishment and "art" work	Introduce girl to cooking, housework, dolls

Chance to dress up and play-act Assumption that he is doing his best in school Pictures and books about history as well as "the facts of life" Sense of belonging in family Discussion of his opinions on menus, vacations, etc. Being read to Contact with culture: museums, films, etc. Reinforcement for acceptable behavior	School-phobia common; do all you can to keep him there Plan "show and tell" for whole family Encourage boy in sports, other masculine activities Assign daily chores: make the bed, feed the pet, do the dishes Allowance (?); help him respect property right of others Ignore "dirty" talk—he's just testing Punish for lying, cheating, stealing

4 ◆◆◆◆◆◆

NIGHTTIME PROBLEMS

"If I could only get one good night's sleep!"

A mother can usually stand a sleepless night or two with her wakeful child if she knows there is an end to it. But she can lose her pleasant perspective if she is faced with repeated sleepless nights after a long day of needling by her child. This night *and* day aggravation will turn the most loving, kind, patient mother into a bear.

Only recently has there been any meaningful research done on sleep. Some scientists now believe that sleep is the natural human state and wakefulness is only a device to allow the body to seek nourishment and excrete wastes. A newborn baby seems to awaken only to eat or have a bowel movement, then goes back to sleep again unless bothered by colic or sickness.

Experts have discovered that we all need to sleep—and dream, for varying amounts of time; that if deprived of our minimum, we become mean, irritable, and occasionally psychotic. Most mothers could have told us so in the first place.

Some areas of the sleeping brain are more responsive than others; that is, a mother may disregard a loud car backfire but leap out of bed when her baby goes "peep." For this and other reasons, there are obvious differences in the amount and the depth of sleep in both children and adults. Children who are active, busy, and growing require deeper and longer sleep. However, there does not seem to be a great correlation between the depth of sleep and daytime activity level. Some babies are so busy when awake that they sleep the sleep of the exhausted. Others, who are nervous and tense, seem to sleep lightly—it does not take much more than a lump in a mattress to drive them wild and keep them awake.

Most babies' sleep needs can be predicted by their behavior in the newborn nursery. The race-horse type of baby is usually touchy, colicky, and a light sleeper. If a touchy woman has this baby as her introduction to motherhood, she may rapidly become unstrung and, of course, further stimulate her sensitive baby. They may both need temporary separation or sedation. On the other hand, if a quick, restless woman brings home the plug-horse variety who needs only a full stomach and a diaper change between long periods of sleep, she may worry that he is anemic, sick, or has a thyroid deficiency.

Nevertheless, most homes and most babies fall somewhere in between these two extremes. A slow, easy-going baby is more likely to be found in a slow, easy-going family. If the home activity level is rather high, then a race-horse type baby might not even be noticed. There is also some evidence that where there are different activity levels under one roof, a compromise is achieved over the years; the fast tend to slow down and the slow tend to speed up. The blood pressures of man and wife are more likely to approximate each other than for one to maintain a high pressure and the other a low one. Similarly, the activity level of any one house rises or falls depending on the amount of noise and liveliness demonstrated by the baby therein. After a while, the baby and parents have lived together long enough to compromise, and everybody gets along quite well.

Somewhere between three weeks and three months, babies who are not diseased or allergic usually begin to sleep about twelve hours at night. The mother who is communicating with her child has a sixth sense about his needs and seems to know automatically whether he needs a nap or a feeding. If he is laughing and smiling more than half the time, he is probably getting adequate rest. If she senses that he is an excitable child, she may find it best to avoid unduly exciting this self-winding organism, and provide him a darkened room with as little noise as possible.

Most babies seem to be able to sleep anywhere, but I assume a firm, nonallergic mattress, a crib large enough to allow some movement, a quiet room, and a temperature of 65° to 70° F. are ideal. Washable synthetic or cotton bedclothes are best. The amount of covering should be that which would be comfortable for an adult. Since the baby's hands and feet tend to feel cold to the touch, feeling his back is a better way to estimate how warm he is. If hot and sweaty, he should have fewer covers or less clothing. Bed toys should be minimal, buttonless, eyeless, washable, and nonallergic; these "security friends" frequently must last for years if the baby gets attached to them. The baby usually decides whether he will sleep on his stomach, back, or side. The only problem is, the prone baby may develop a pigeon-toed tendency if he sleeps in the knee-chest position. (Check with your doctor.)

One of our colicky babies slept better in a semisitting position; he could burp, breathe, pass gas, or do *something* better this way. Some babies go to sleep more readily if, after a bottle and a good burp, they are placed in bed supine and are fed another ounce as they slowly pass out.

Babies fuss or cry if they are hungry, thirsty, or tired; and a mother can sense what the trouble is. But if it is your first baby in the house and you are not used to his noises, in the first few weeks you may not be able to differentiate whether he is in pain or just needs to cry a little bit or be active. About 50 percent of babies cry themselves to sleep, and you may have to experiment: Pick him up? Rock him? Feed him again? Offer a pacifier? If baby is full and has been changed and is not sick, you should put him into bed with a gentle pat and a cheerful, "See you tomorrow."

If you are a good actress, you can pull off this trick and may not be bothered again until breakfast. By the time you get around to the second or third baby, there may be so much noise in the house that you will not hear the newcomer's crying or fussing. Frequently, when you have finally heard the cry and are ready to feed him, he will have gone back to sleep, assuming perhaps that no one was going to feed him and there was nothing better to do.

Most mothers can tolerate about twenty minutes of crying. It seems to me this is the cutoff point. If baby *has* to cry himself to sleep, fifteen or twenty minutes should do it! If he's crying after this, he must be refed, changed, burped; something must be wrong. Some babies, if they cry longer than this, become hysterical and continue to cry because they are crying. (Again, the vicious cycle.) Some have such a good gag reflex that they vomit and have to be refed.

Initially, though, you should steel yourself to this twenty minutes of anguish. If you pick him up after five minutes of crying because you couldn't wait through the twenty, you just may excite him more—and he may come to expect this at bedtime. It is easier to prevent the routine of lying down with a baby to get him to sleep in the first year than to try to stop this when it's become a fixed habit at the age of two to four years.

Some babies are full of milk, burped, and all set to go right off to sleep, but apparently they didn't get enough sucking pleasure. If they have not found their thumb yet, then the lesser of the two evils, the pacifier,* is justified. These kids seem very much like the orally-oriented gentleman who must have his after-dinner glass of port and a cigar to help his digestion. If you find no other good way to get your baby to sleep, then you are justified in trying the pacifier. After all, later on in life—and hopefully before the age of five—you can hide this device from your child much more easily than you can his thumb.

One of our children continued to awaken us at night, so at five months we put her in a separate room. Either she did not hear our snoring or she stopped "asking" for us because we were out of sight and not so readily available to respond to her every whimper. In any case, all went well.

Once baby and mother compromise with each other's routine demands, going to bed at night is no big problem until the age of seven months. At this time, as mentioned in the previous chapter, the baby begins to realize that he's not attached to his mother by some magical umbilical cord. When put to bed at night, he begins to scream. Often he is able to stand up and grab hold of the crib sides, and then seems unable to let himself down. He really is hysterical. The normal mother's reflex is to go in, pick

---

* The Nuk pacifier, which is imported from Germany, fits the mouth and gums better than others. Most stores carry them.

him up, soothe him, and put him down again. The wise mother does no more than this, and she does not allow her child to get any great satisfaction out of this routine except the reassurance that he is all right. She is supposed to be gentle but firm, put him down in his bed, turn out the light, and leave, holding her head up high and knowing that this is the last time she will have to come in. (It usually isn't, however.) But if she takes the child out of bed and into another part of the house, the child gets to expect this routine. Each succeeding night the bedtime routine becomes that much more difficult.

Unless your child gets so hysterical and sick that he vomits, it is really better for you to put him down and let him scream it out for himself. The main way to reassure him, of course, is to be there the next morning. Finally, after weeks of screaming at night for one to four hours, the child senses that everything is all right because you are always there the next day. He usually drops his protests because they haven't done him any good, and he will accept whatever bedtime hour you have established. After all, you know when your baby is tired and ready to go to sleep. This system is supposed to teach him patience, tolerance, and impulse control—good adult attributes.

Length of sleep varies greatly in babies, but the average infant from three to ten months naps one to two hours in the morning. He will eat lunch, nap another one or two hours in the afternoon, eat supper, then sleep ten to twelve hours at night. After this age, he will sometimes continue the naps, but usually begin his day at a progressively earlier hour. His total sleep time is less, but he disregards household wishes. A clever mother postpones his morning nap by a half hour, offers an early lunch, and combines his two naps into one, thus effectively shortening daytime sleep. Hopefully, this reschedules his morning reveille to a more suitable time. Some babies can be awakened early in the afternoon if they are not too irritable, and will go to bed at a decent time or sleep later the next morning.

The next period of sleep resistance begins close to the age of two. By this time, your child has learned to climb over the side of the crib and come on out to where the action is. You know he is tired and you cannot understand why he does not pop right off to sleep. The two-year-old almost seems to know that once he puts his head down and shuts his eyes, he will sleep. So he sings, cries, fools around, gets out his toys, looks out the window, talks to his hands—anything to keep himself awake, as if he is afraid of missing some big party he thinks is going on in the living room. Father puts him to bed; mother and even grandmother put him to bed; spankings, scoldings, rewards, and stories are tried; *nothing* seems to work. But be stout of heart, firm of purpose. Knowing that your child is tired, leave him in there. Keep the room as free of stimulating toys as possible; he may hurt himself in a dark, cluttered room. You can try fixing up the room like a padded cell—the mattress on the floor (which may preclude falling out of bed), the child, and nothing else. The door is shut firmly but not locked, in case of fire, and a night-light is kept in his room in case he is afraid of the dark. Hopefully, he will become bored and fall asleep. When you hear no more thumping around, you may then tiptoe in and replace him on the mattress if you want to. I would not condemn people who turn the crib or playpen upside down on the mattress, so their child is essentially behind bars. During the day this seems a little harsh, but rightfully confines him at night, especially if he is accident-prone.

Medication for the sleep-resistant child is occasionally a must —to preserve parental sanity. The usual soporific (barbiturate) frequently has just the opposite effect and only stimulates the child or just makes him uncoordinated. He staggers around as if drunk and frequently falls and hurts himself. The tranquilizers and some antihistamines—with their drowsy side effects—are safer. They encourage the child to just put his head down for a minute, often all that is needed for him to drop off to sleep. If a child between the years of three and five still has great reluctance about going to sleep, it usually means that somebody's mishandled his bedtime problem before, or that he is really insecure, fearing that if he doesn't stay awake his home will collapse. Most two- to five-year-olds need twelve hours sleep at night plus a nap of one to three hours. Yet others need no nap, go to bed at nine and are up and cheerful at six. Morning behavior usually indicates whether the previous night's sleep was adequate. Some who cannot sleep need a quiet time in the afternoon in a darkened room, and later at night a bed-oriented book or game before going to sleep. Others have to rock the bed for a while, suck their thumb, twist their hair, rub a blanket on their nose, or indulge in some sort of nesting-type behavior. Don't force the child to stop these activities unless you have a satisfactory and acceptable (to him, that is) substitute.

Bedtime should be a cozy, warm, friendly, secure time. Too often it is a hurried, tense, "march off to bed, shut your eyes, shut up, and go to sleep or I'll smack you," time. Carefully planned stalling actions are common, such as the final bathroom trip, the forgotten toothbrushing, prayers with interminable "God bless Uncle Ed's," putting Pooh Bear to bed, requests to adjust window shades and blankets. "Read the story again" and "Scratch my back" can go on forever. Depending on the child, some time limit should be set. But bedtime is an ideal interlude to set aside for a little conversation. A few peaceful bedtime moments spent with your child when he is small will lessen embarrassment of approaching him later in adolescence when you feel the need for a meaningful talk.

The bed in which we spend about one-third of our lives should be large, firm, and clean. Sleep is best done singly. It should be in a quiet room where one may have private, profound, important thoughts.

A tired child may go to sleep, seem secure and relaxed, but wake up a few hours later. The trouble here, of course, is that he has been refreshed by his rest and nothing seems to put him back to sleep again. Any number of things can wake him up. In early infancy, perhaps the most common cause is hunger. After six or eight months this is no longer a problem. It may be teething (but this is unusual) or an ear infection, In a boy, a very common cause of wakefulness is an ammonia burn causing a slight ulceration just inside the opening of the end of the penis. As the salty urine goes over this area it stings, burns, and awakens him. Obviously, the trick is to get rid of the ammonia. One such remedy is listed under "ammoniacal diaper" in the "Conditions" section of the "Quick Reference Directory."

Just the act of urinating wakes many babies, especially the boy whose penis is in contact with a lot of salty urine at three in the morning. Once eight or ten months have gone by, an effort can be made to cut down the amount of fluid and milk he is drinking. Fill him up with solids so he will drink less milk and urinate less to create less ammonia. If he urinates three or four times a day, he does not need extra fluid.

Another common reason for abbreviated sleep is a gas pain or cramp caused by something your child ate for supper. The more common irritants are fish, pork, corn, green vegetables, and wheat. You will already be aware of a milk allergy, since your child's diet was largely milk in the first several months of life. If he was a good sleeper when mainly on milk and developed a gas problem later, then a recent addition to his diet might be to blame. Parents forget that anything made from flour—teething biscuits, cookies, toast, bread, and crackers—all contain wheat and can cause gas, cramps, diarrhea, and often a redness around the anal opening. The usual diaper rash from ammonia or citrus would be on whatever area the urine touches, but usually *not* between the buttocks, because urine rarely gets in there. If redness is confined to the anal opening, it suggests that your child is eating some solid food that is disturbing him. The food that is giving him rashes may also be giving him gas, which wakes him up at night.

When your child is two or three years old, the most common cause of night wakefulness is pinworms. One of my four-month-old patients acquired worms from his four-year-old sister who was "helpful" in feeding and changing him. (A child does not develop worms without someone to act as carrier.) The mother thought her baby had colic, but one day when she was changing his diaper he happened to discharge a stool with a great number of quarter-inch white, crawly, squirming worms. His mother screamed and ran for the phone. We treated both children with the appropriate medicine, and both were soon cheerful and happy.

In infant girls, I have seen these small worms migrate forward into the vaginal opening. I have read of rare cases where they continued on into the bladder and ureters into the kidney. Or, again in the case of girls, into the vagina, through the uterus, out the fallopian tubes, and into the peritoneum. This seems fantastic, but it does happen! A large series of studies indicate that worms can obstruct the appendix, causing appendicitis. Pathologists are no longer surprised to find segments of worms in an infected appendix—and not just pinworms either. Many other kinds of worms afflict humans, from fishworms to tapeworms to long roundworms. But in children, the most common is the pinworm.

The pinworm's life cycle works somewhat like this: The pregnant female worms come out at night to lay their microscopic eggs around the anal opening. Each female may lay several thousand. This causes intense itching; the child usually scratches this area, picking up a number of eggs underneath his fingernails. He may be bathed daily and his fingernails may be short and clean, but he will still harbor some eggs under his nails. Then when he handles books, toys, or athletic equipment, he leaves some of these eggs behind. Another child may pick up these toys and, of course, transmit the eggs from his hand to his mouth. It does not take more than two eggs (one male, one female) to start a new cycle in a new child. When these eggs get to the colon they hatch, and male meets female and female gets pregnant. Out she goes like a good mother and lays her thousand eggs outside the anal opening. Again the itch, and again the cycle is repeated.

The cardinal symptom of worms is night wakefulness. If a child is wakeful at night and not sick with sore throat, ear infection, or gas attack, he may have worms. Other worm symptoms to check for are stomachaches, teeth grinding, and an itchy, burning sensation around the anal opening. Most afflicted children are also irritable and tense because they have not been sleeping properly. They cry easily, are grouchy, fussy, and often mean. These symptoms might ordinarily point to a behavior problem, but before calling the child psychologist, try treating your child for worms. Most remedies are now quite effective, and within seventy-two hours after the proper dose, your child should have been relieved of enough of his internal population to show noticeable improvement.

Some doctors refuse to treat for worms unless they see them. They may ask the mother to bring in a sample of her child's stool or a piece of transparent tape that she has pushed against the anal opening, thus perhaps picking up minute eggs that the doctor can examine under the microscope. It seems quite ridiculous to go through all this. If the child has worm symptoms and has not had adequate treatment for them for a few months, he should be treated on the assumption that he has them again. The treatment will not hurt him in any case. Two or three effective medicines are available by prescription. One dose is given by mouth and repeated in ten days. It only kills the adult worms, so the repeat dose is needed to kill those that have developed from the eggs present ten days previously. Side effects from the medicine are rare and no enemas are necessary.

Once and for all, I would like to dispel a number of old wives' tales on the subject.

(1) Worms are not universally found in the poor or the dirty, but in all strata of society, though unsanitary habits certainly encourage them.

(2) Sitting on cold cement does not cause worms.

(3) Neither does eating candy.

(4) A huge appetite is not a symptom of worms. When afflicted with any type of worm, the victim usually has a poor appetite.

(5) A child who picks his nose does not do so because he has worms. But, the child who picks his nose or sucks his thumb is more likely to wind up with some worm eggs because he always has his hand in his face.

Almost every day a mother calls me about her child's worms. Some authorities feel that upwards of 60 percent of all children have them at one time or another. Pinworms are more common in some areas of the country (such as the deep South) than in others. Until recently, they were considered to be signs of poor care and an unclean home. Anybody with worms was automatically of a lower social order and obviously did not bathe regularly. Even today, the general public does not hear about worms, because when a horrified mother discovers that *her* child has them, she seldom broadcasts the news.

This attitude echoes the teaching that we had in medical school: Only a "certain type of person" gets worms, and if you washed regularly and kept reasonably neat toilet habits, you would never be afflicted. However, the worms have proved us all wrong by being found in the cleanest homes as well as the dirtiest. I have developed a new theory (perhaps based mainly on the fact that my own children have had worms periodically): Children have worms because they have friends. If a child does not socialize too well, he may not have any friends from whom to get worms. So I would say, if your child gets worms frequently, he may be just "relating to his peers." (If he *never* gets worms, he either has antisocial tendencies or uninfected classmates.)

Some form of controlled medication in the classroom seems prudent. There is no reason why the children who are usually playing and exchanging toys, books, and worm eggs with each other could not all be treated together. If a whole school class or neighborhood, city or county (ideally, the whole world) could be treated at one time, we might be able to get rid of these pesky creatures and stop their cycle. Pinworms are really a social disease among children. However, because of the widespread but mistaken belief that worms are the product of dirty and inadequate home care, most mothers treat their children in secrecy, without letting school or neighbors know what they are doing. Thus, by the time a mother has her child free of worms, those defunct worms' grandchildren are incubating in her neighbor's child, who in a couple of weeks will be ready to give his worm eggs back to their original donor.

Often a child with worms will wake up screaming with terrible nightmares. I think worms irritate a child so that he is more likely to dream, and of course he does not dream about worms. He has to have some content for his dreams, so he will be dreaming about the last thing he remembers—usually the horror show he watched on television. TV gets blamed for a lot of symptoms that are really due to worms, so before you pull down your antenna, try a visit to the doctor.

Actually, dreams are considered devices to keep the sleeper from waking up. Even while asleep, a child's brain picks up little noises that ordinarily would disturb him enough to make him restless. But his imagination "explains" them away through a dream. Thus a cat-fight outside his window becomes a jungle safari where he is stalking tigers in the bush. Dreams are also a medium to hash out tensions and desires accumulated during the day, and, as such, are quite essential. A person allowed to sleep enough but awakened whenever he starts to dream will become agitated and disturbed. Various stimuli from the body may also influence the brain and cause more and increasingly vivid dreams. Of course, if the jungle safari gets out of control and becomes a nightmare, the sufferer may awaken frightened. There are psychiatric reasons for nightmares, but in children, physical causes head the list. A sickness with fever makes many children have delirious dreams or have night terrors—it usually takes thirty minutes to fully awaken the child who has frantically cried out. He is disoriented; he continues to call for his mother even though she is right there trying to soothe him.

If a child has difficulty going to sleep after age five, he usually has an emotional problem, a feeling of insecurity or overwhelming panic that prevents him from relaxing. But, if he goes to sleep fairly readily and *then* awakens, pinworms, stomachaches, or urinary problems would seem more likely.

One condition difficult to diagnose is the nighttime seizure. These seizures are a form of epilepsy and fortunately are rare. We know from studies of brain-wave patterns of people in normal sleep that when we go from one phase to another, different brain patterns are observed. A person may have one area of his brain that is susceptible to overstimulation. This "irritable focus" might be triggered to discharge powerful electrical impulses, in a way analogous to a short circuit. If surrounding areas of the brain are relatively quiet, the resulting "current" may not be contained and spreads to other areas of the brain, thus starting a seizure.

Unless someone is observing the victim in his sleep, the true nature of this "attack" will not be discovered. Sometimes a child will awaken from a frightening dream covered with perspiration. He may have urinated or lost his stool. He may feel exhausted or have a bad headache. This could imply that he had a spell. If a child who has been recently treated for worms awakens at night and seems frightened or not in control of his faculties, then I would assume he had most likely suffered some type of seizure. An effort should be made to rule this out by appropriate brain-wave tests.

Again, nocturnal seizures are rare, but many go unrecognized. They may or may not be associated with daytime attacks. Medication helps, and perhaps if the victim is not afflicted during the day, his medicine might be given more appropriately at bedtime so as to have its maximum effect during the sleeping hours. The small percentage of people who wet the bed during a seizure are often erroneously diagnosed as having a psychiatric problem. Seizures in children can disappear at maturity, but medicine seems to improve control and "cure" rates.

There are many harmless but aggravating things children do in their sleep—teeth-grinding, head knocking, and so on. These activities bother the adults in the house, but apparently not the performer, who seems content and rested during the day. Such actions should be tolerated as sleep-savers because, if curtailed, the child usually awakens. Thumb-sucking can be noisy but is better than smoking in bed. Sleep-walking can be dangerous, and warning bells or lights might best be devised to alert *you*—the sleepwalker should be awakened gradually. Bed-rocking may serve some useful purpose to the sleeper, but tenants on the floor below are not interested in deducing his motives. Placing the mattress on the floor deadens the sound and keeps the bed from being demolished.

However, by far the most irritating, frustrating thing a child can do is to wet the bed. It is hard *not* to punish him for his smelly, sodden mess; it is difficult to believe he cannot help it. The children I have mentioned previously sleep lightly or not enough, but the enuretic (bed-wetting) child seems to be *too* sound a sleeper. He is too conked out to sense that his bladder is full, which would rouse a lighter sleeper to get up and do something about it. Such a child may even dream he is respectably using the toilet. (Again, the dream serves as a device to help him stay asleep.)

By definition, an enuretic child is any girl over age four, or any boy over age five, who wets the bed. This can occur from one to ten times a night. There are as many theories as to causes as there are to cures (most of which are fruitless). Emotional problems can be a reason. "Passive aggression" is the psychiatrist's term, usually applied to a boy who resents his parents for some real or imagined insult. Unable to externalize or verbalize his aggression, he subconsciously bed-wets as a means of getting even. "Urethral aggression" is another, perhaps less savory term for this syndrome.

Genetic or inherited factors are felt to be the most common cause of bed-wetting (accounting for 80 percent). In the remaining 20 percent, the culprits include drinking too many fluids after four o'clock in the afternoon, allergies, structural abnormalities of the urinary system, and abnormal brain-wave patterns (the child who has a seizure when maverick nerve impulses stimulate the bladder muscle).

When a mother realizes that her child is a bed-wetter, the first thing she should do is have her doctor make a routine urinalysis to search for albumen, sugar, and pus cells. A normal urinalysis does not necessarily rule out structural anomalies. Some children have double kidneys. All sorts of oddities may occur in a child who appears healthy. If these are suspected, X-rays and perhaps a specialist are needed to determine the size and efficiency of the bladder and kidneys. In a new technique, an X-ray–opaque dye is concentrated in the kidneys and flows down through the ureters into the bladder, thus giving a clear picture of these soft organs. Sometimes the urologist uses a cystoscope to look inside the bladder for defects in valves and tubing. If urine is not being excreted properly or completely, it is likely to become infected, like stagnant water. Thus, if a bed-wetter has had a number of bladder or kidney infections, some structural deviation is usually present.

Some estimate of urinary health can be made by watching the child urinate. Without straining, the stream should be forceful, making bubbles in the toilet bowl. The stream size is important. A child who wets frequently during the day with poor control and constant dribbling should be investigated by a urologist. It can occasionally mean some nervous instability of the bladder or an allergic problem.

Because bed-wetting is reasonably rare in the female, and much more common in the male, a more extensive investigation is necessary when the patient is a girl. She might be more likely to have a structural abnormality. Obviously, any child should be investigated for other systemic conditions such as tuberculosis, anemia, diabetes, and rheumatic fever that may play a small role in bed-wetting. If the child is not feeling well generally, this could affect the urinary functions.

If the child still bed-wets after structural anomalies are ruled out and chronic infections cleared up, then consider an allergy. Perhaps one out of twenty children will wet the bed for this reason—it is as if their bladder were sneezing. A urinary allergy is usually related to something fluid in the child's diet, such as milk or orange juice, but it could conceivably come from chocolate, tomatoes, pineapples, or peaches. *What*, rather than *how much*, seems to irritate the bladder to push out urine at undesirable times. A child may be labeled a neurotic because he wets the bed, but his "neurosis" is cured when he forgets his evening milk.

If you suspect milk allergy, cut out milk, ice cream, and cottage cheese from his diet for one day. If he stays dry, milk is the culprit, and without it his bed-wetting days are over.

Many emotionally disturbed children wet the bed, but not all bed-wetters are neurotic or unhappy. After a child passes the age of six or seven he usually becomes embarrassed about his condition, especially when he finds that he cannot spend the night with friends or go on camping trips. His mother is also getting discouraged. Her efforts to get him up at night, restrict his fluids, and un-deprive him emotionally (if that is her working theory), have all come to naught. She often cannot conceal her disgust. Then, perhaps *because* he is wetting the bed, he may get neurotic or feel inferior or develop emotional problems that come as a *result* of the bed-wetting. So, when psychologists see a withdrawn child who is wetting the bed, it is frequently impossible for them to decide which condition came first, the bed-wetting or the emotional problem.

The child with a familial or inherited trait for enuresis, besides being a deep sleeper, usually has a small or "immature" bladder. His kidneys are fine, but his bladder is not able to store all the urine that has accumulated during the night. His bladder sends a message to the spinal cord saying it is full. But no message from the spinal cord comes to the social part of the brain that knows it is not acceptable to urinate in bed because Mother will get mad. It is as if the connections in the switchboard up in the brain were asleep and no message could get through from down below. The spinal cord does not have any social awareness, so without the brain telling it what to do, it acts on its own authority. It sends back the message to the bladder, "Dump it!" The bladder is properly formed, but the sphincter muscle designed to hold in the urine cannot seem to withstand the bladder wall's strong muscles.

The treatment for this frustrating condition is not universally satisfactory. All doctors have seen many bed-wetting patients. After ruling out anatomical abnormalities and allergies affecting the urinary tract, the first question is, "Is there a family history of this condition?" In many cases, the mother will admit that she had a couple of brothers and a father who wet the bed, but that she didn't. She usually doesn't know of any history of bed-wetting on her husband's side of the family. Few husbands, of course, want their wives to know that they were less than perfect males, and wet the bed as a child.

My father, the doctor, had a son and a grandson who were less than perfect in that respect. Whenever patients came to him with the bed-wetting problem, he would say, "If you find something that works, let me know. I'd like to try it at home." Most doctors "solve" the problem by saying, "He will outgrow it."

However, when bed-wetters outgrow the problem and later are saddled with children in the same fix, they usually react excessively because they don't like to see their own "forgotten" weakness showing up again. This seems to be a natural response, but only serves to aggravate the condition. Placing so much emotional emphasis on this one symptom almost always serves to make it worse. Many children seem to continue bed-wetting on purpose as if they knew it aggravated their parents.

Today, when so many remedies are available for so many other conditions, we doctors are embarrassed to say, "Sorry." We attempt treatment without raising false hopes of rapid cures. We play down the condition and provide reassurance. We try to get the mother to accept her child and stop nagging and punishing him for this unconscious act. There is no way to punish the unconscious ganglia of a child's nervous system.

Almost all children outgrow the condition when they fully mature. Their muscle strength is greater, their bladder capacity has increased, and they may not be sleeping as deeply as they did in their childhood—they become more aware of the full bladder impulses that suggest to the sleeping brain to do something about going to the bathroom.

Many way-out home remedies have been successful because they are tried at the time the child was destined to outgrow the problem. Some may work for the wrong reasons. One ridiculous theory holds that if the child sleeps in a head-down position, his liver and intestines will not push on the bladder and incite him to wet his bed. Another states that if the bed creates pressure on the kidneys, they produce more urine, as if they were sponges being squeezed. To counteract this, a board, log, or rock is taped to the child's back to preclude sleep in the supine position. (In both these uncomfortable positions he would not sleep as soundly and may be be more aware when his bladder is full.) Yet an-

other belief has it that salt, salty peanuts, and raisins given at bedtime soak up fluid in the intestinal tract so that there is less urine
secreted by the kidneys. (Most of these drying-up methods only
serve to make the child thirsty—perhaps he will get up for a drink
of water because of his thirst and remember to empty his bladder at the same time.)

The above treatments are quite naive, but if the bed remains
dry, they work.

Many gadgets have been invented that are a little more scientific. One that seems not too inappropriate for males is a sponge-
rubber clothespin device that clamps on the penis. When the boy
starts to urinate in his sleep, the urinary stream hits the clamp.
This hurts. He awakens, removes the clamp, and finishes the job
in the appropriate place. Another device is called the "motor-
man's friend," in which rubber tubing runs from the penis to an
inflatable bladder that can be strapped to the child's leg. This
only serves to catch the urine. The child sleeps through the night,
but the bed is dry and the smell less.

The most reliable device, recommended by authorities medical
and nonmedical, is a wire mesh underneath the bed sheet. When
the salt urine comes into contact with this, an electric circuit is
closed and a light and/or buzzer is activated. Hopefully, the child
awakens before he is finished emptying his bladder, and may
eventually learn to awaken at the time of urination. (It is a condi-
tioned reflex, such as the response of Pavlov's dog who salivated
when he heard the bell.) Under proper supervision, this method
has been about 80 percent successful. Depending on how accurate the reports are, it may approach a 100 percent cure rate.
(The family's interest and the child's motivation are as important
as the device.) Of course, physical conditions and structural
anomalies have to be ruled out before either cure would be
effective.

Because doctors did not invent these machines, they are sometimes loath to use them—they seem like a form of cheating. But
doctors *are* trained to use medicines, and recently a number of
drugs have been found to have an apparent effect on bed-wetting. All of these medicines belong to the group called imipramine. When given in appropriate doses, imipramines will help
control more than 50 percent of bed-wetters. Treatment may be
as simple as giving this medicine at bedtime. Sometimes, after

several weeks of drug-induced dryness, it seems that a bladder habit is established that continues when the medicine is withdrawn. Imipramines seem to be safe, but should be given under a doctor's supervision.

A logical training regimen can help supplement the above treatment, providing the child is at least seven years old and motivated. During the day he can be rewarded for holding his urine instead of passing it at the first urge. He should also learn to stop and start the stream a few times during urination. These exercises can stretch his bladder capacity and develop voluntary brain control over the sphincter purse-string muscle that holds urine in the bladder. Presently I favor medicines as the first, most convenient, and inexpensive method. Failing these, the electric devices should be tried.

As with so many other children's problems, the family's attitude is all-important. A casual, relaxed approach to bed-wetting is much better than the frantic, "We-are-going-to-do-something-right-this-minute," clenched-teeth attitude. If the child has wet himself every night since birth, he is most probably afflicted with the more common "immature bladder" that tends to run in families. If, however, he develops this trait after the age of three or four, you should look for physical problems, diseases, and more importantly, school pressures or other emotional difficulties that may have cropped up while you were not looking.

After a few years, most parents find they have gotten use to their child's nocturnal idiosyncrasies. They have learned to nap or get by with less sleep, or somehow compromise with their child's unchangeable sleep patterns. Then they are kept awake by their *own* problems—gas, arthritis, cold feet, drafts, snoring spouses, or worries about their adolescent's behavior. Few alarm clocks are needed by parents of growing children.

SLEEP RESISTANCE AND NIGHT WAKEFULNESS
Possible Causes

Age	Won't Go to Sleep	Awakens after Going to Sleep
Birth to 6 Months	Hunger Colic Over stimulation	Hunger; Colic; lost pacifier; too small bed; sickness, earache; cutting teeth; urine contacting open sores; urinary infection
6 Months to 15 Months	Over stimulation Fear of separation "Spoiled" (?) Nap too long	Ear infection; fever; pinworms; diaper rash; gas from food; croup; allergy to pillow, blanket, or toy
15 Months to 3 Years	Playing a "game" Anxiety, fear of separation Nap too long	Pinworms; diaper rash; sickness; teething; bed too small; refused to have bowel movement during day, relaxes and has it at night
3 to 5 Years	Nap too long Overstimulated. Spoiled? No rules "Ghosts" or "snakes" in room Family arguments in next room	Pinworms; sickness; fall out of bed
5 Years on	Doesn't need so much sleep Parents fighting House too noisy	Pinworms; sickness; full bladder; seizure

5 ❦❦❦❦

THE HYPERMOTOR CHILD

"He can't seem to sit still for a minute."

By far the childhood condition most commonly mistaken for a psychiatric problem is that suffered by the hypermotor child. A victim of this problem has a short attention span, is distractible, and overly active. He seems to be driven. He is a constant aggravation, either physically or verbally; he disrupts the home and the school. Because he is such an obvious disturbance, mothers and teachers try to control him. But he always seems to get even more upset by their methods, and soon he develops various secondary emotional problems. It bothers me that so few doctors, educators, and psychologists know how to treat this condition—especially since medical literature has been pointing out effective medicines for it ever since 1937.

Dr. Charles Bradley, a pediatrician and psychiatrist in Portland, Oregon, has written many fine medical articles describing the diagnosis and treatment of hypermotor children. His lines of communication to the various medical, paramedical, and educational fields have somehow not been operating. I am in debt to Dr. Bradley's work for my discussion of this neglected childhood problem.

When I speak to parent-teacher groups and mention just one

example of hypermotor behavior in the classroom, I begin to see nods of agreement from the teachers. When I talk about hypermotor behavior in the home, certain mothers seem to feel that I have their living rooms bugged. Let me start here by describing a classroom scene.

The setting is the first-grade classroom of any school in early September. The teacher has gotten the children in their seats and is trying to remember names. In many of the students she notices the usual nervousness, tears, and shyness. But one boy, John, seems to be more restless than the others. She finds him up and out of his seat to ask a question at the slightest—or no—provocation. If someone drops a pencil, he is right over there to pick it up. If a car goes by outside, he rushes to the window and points it out to the rest of the class. Despite the teacher's insistence that he stay in his seat, he seems physically unable to do so. When the principal comes to the door to check on the classroom, John is, of course, the first one out of his seat and off to the door to see him.

"Hi, there!" he says. "Come in. We're having class."

The principal looks at the teacher with one eyebrow raised as if to say, "What's the matter, don't you have this boy in control? Aren't you motivating him properly? Why won't he stay in his seat?"

The teacher looks back at the principal with a half smile and shrugs her shoulders a little bit as if to say, "I've tried, but what can I do?"

So, by the time ten o'clock has rolled around, the teacher and the principal are calling his mother.

Strangely enough, his mother is expecting the call. This is the first time in six years that she has been able to sit down quietly after breakfast and drink an unspilled cup of coffee. She knew something was wrong; it was *too* quiet.

"You have a nice boy," says the principal on the phone. "However, we have found him seriously lacking in self-control. He's immature. He's out of his seat all the time. He's a disturbance to the class, and if his behavior doesn't improve you'll have to keep him home another year. Maybe we'll try the first grade over again next year." The mother is crushed, but not surprised. During all those six years of discipline and home care, she knew she had no real control over her son. She hoped that school would be the best answer—she felt that teachers must have other children like John and would know how to control him. However, now the school feels that *she* should have been able to teach John how to control himself. So, in effect, the school blames Mother and Mother blames the school—the lack of communication between these two is often phenomenal.

Now the child I have described is characterized by two unforgettable features: (1) He has a short attention span, and (2) he is distractible. A number of other things may characterize this boy. He may have behavior problems. Reading is his worst subject; physical education is his best. His emotions are usually labile —that is, he laughs and cries easily. But mainly, he is hypermotor: extremely active physically, unable to sit still long enough to accomplish the work he is supposed to do. He's smart enough to do the work required, but he will not put it down on paper so that it can be graded. His teacher usually feels that he is an underachiever.

Of course, this is not just something that began in September when he was six years old and started the first grade. He has been this way since birth, and was only aggravated by the sights and sounds of the classroom. His mother will remember he was always a poor sleeper; he may have had colic, and in general, was a fussy baby. He sometimes awoke early. He was often accident-prone, climbing up on things only to fall off. He seemed to have to be busy. He understood dangers when they were explained to him, but still would have to see for himself. He had to keep testing gravity, for instance, by falling many times. He sometimes got in his parents' pills and medicines. He may have run away from home. He often ran into the street. He usually lacked fear, and ordinary discipline did not seem to have any effect.

Many such children grow up to be perfectly normal. In fact, the average two-year-old is distractible and has a short attention span, but when these two symptoms persist up to the age of six they are often considered signs of immaturity. Such a child's intelligence seems all right, but his emotions and behavior are immature; he continues to act like a two-year-old.

He can really be a pain in the neck. "What's for lunch?" he asks.

"I don't know what's for lunch," Mother says. "I haven't finished cooking breakfast yet."

"What's for supper then?" he asks.

"Eeeeaaaugh!" she groans.

The interest in food is understandable. Most hyperactive children burn up so many calories racing their engines that they eat tremendous amounts, but stay thin and wiry. Some, however, get their caloric needs by eating small amounts all day—their short attention span does not allow them to sit down to a meal for more than thirty seconds at a time. Some do better if fed by themselves; they get too stimulated by the others at the table.

Many mothers feel that it is somehow their fault that their child got this way. Some think that the child has picked up their own nervous, restless tendencies. I have found, however, that the reverse is more likely true. An accident-prone child who is into everything, constantly active, and pestering his mother twenty-four hours a day can only make her nervous.

Her tired husband, home from his labors, usually punishes the child after she has read the grievance list for the day. Dinner is a shambles, and bedtime yet another battle. When friends come over to have a cup of coffee, they see this child tearing around the house and they assume his anxious, distraught mother started the problem. The neighbors do not know what the mother was like before she had her child. She might have been the most happily relaxed person in the world. *He* started it.

Any teacher who has read this description will be able to recognize the hypermotor child. I am sure most teachers will be able to name such a child in their class right now. If you want a volunteer to take a message to the office, he is the first one up in the front to say, "I'll go, I'll go." So the teacher sends the child with some message to the office, hoping he will use up some extra energy. And within seconds it seems the child is back in the room again.

"I delivered that. What'll I do now?"

"Just stay in your seat," the teacher says. But he cannot do so. He is hyperactive; his battery is overcharged.

The child is better off if he is somewhat isolated from the rest of the class. So she tries to put him up next to her desk or in a corner behind a shelf. But he is unable to disregard unimportant stimuli, is distracted if anyone else sneezes, shuffles his feet, sharpens a pencil, or turns the pages of a book. This quality may persist for years. Now, in the first conference that the teacher has with the parents (if the child has not already been sent home and told that he cannot come back until a year has gone by), the teacher tells his mother that he is creating problems in the classroom.

"I think there may be something wrong with your child," the teacher says, somewhat embarrassed to even bring it up. "He has trouble getting his work finished. He has trouble staying in his seat. He has a short attention span."

The most difficult and important thing a teacher has to do is get this message across to the mother. Communication is often difficult, because a mother feels that any criticism of her child is criticism of herself, and she goes on the defensive. But in this case she is not at fault—she has done her level best, but so has the teacher. Nevertheless, the mother assumes that she has not taught the child self-control, so she says, "What are we going to do?"

"Why don't you take the child to the doctor?" The mother agrees.

When this child is in the doctor's office, he is alone with his mother and the doctor—there are no distracting stimuli such as there are in the classroom. He has nothing terribly wrong with him. His tonsils may be slightly enlarged, he may have a little wax in his ears, his feet may be a little flat, and his shoulders droop a bit. But his heart is beating, his lungs are clear, and there is no source of infection. The doctor may even check his blood and find he is not anemic, that the child's teeth are not greatly decayed, his hearing and vision are normal. In short, he is an average six-year-old, so the doctor asks, "What seems to be the problem?"

"Well," the mother says, "I don't know. They can't seem to teach him anything in school. I know he's a bright boy, but they say he won't stay in his seat and put the work down on paper. What are we going to do, Doctor?"

The doctor pats the boy on the shoulder and reassures her by stating, "He's a fine boy and there's nothing wrong with him. I'm sure his intelligence is all right. You take him back and tell his teacher she ought to be able to teach him just beautifully."

That does it! Now armed with a scientific pronouncement, the mother pushes the boy back into the classroom, turns to the teacher defiantly, and says, "I took him to the doctor and he says he's okay. If you can't teach him, there's something wrong with you."

If the teacher can get the message over to 80 or 90 percent of her first-grade class, then she assumes she is doing quite a good job. But she has never been sure that her teaching techniques were *that* perfect. So her head droops and, feeling guilty, she agrees to take the child back and give him special attention. But the problem is still there. Even if the teacher stands behind the child holding his head toward the book or the paper in an effort to make him concentrate, none of her motivational techniques will work.

The doctor finds nothing wrong, because there is no test that can really *prove* any particular child is hypermotor. The doctor wants to make the diagnosis himself; he is upset if somebody else has to make it for him. He may ask the psychologists to give him some help, and they find that the child has an average IQ. But again, no specific psychological test will indicate that a boy has this abnormality.

The point I am trying to make is that the *teacher* has to diagnose this condition. She has twenty or thirty other children in the class. If this one child, John, stands out so obviously, the teacher is the one who is supposed to communicate this to his mother and make it stick. The mother is supposed to have enough rapport with the doctor to be able to call him and say, "You know my son John. He's always been a busy, accident-prone child. Now the teacher says he's distractible and hypermotor, and has a short attention span. She says you can do something."

And, indeed, the teacher is right. There is no point in the doctor saying, "He will outgrow it." We know that most hypermotor children do, but something has to be done right now, while John is still six years old. He can be helped by medication, and there is no reason why it should be withheld.

In addition to a teacher's evaluation, there are many things a doctor can look for to help him decide whether the condition exists. Psychologists can help a bit. They have found that many children who have suffered a slight hurt to the nervous system earlier in life get better verbal scores than performance scores on intelligence tests. If there is a wide scatter between these two scores, it is a possible indication of some hurt to the nervous system, even though there does not seem to be any neurological test to confirm this. Some hypermotor children also have a slight tremor, some have some hyperactive reflexes, some do not have a visual afterimage when they shut their eyes after looking at a bright light. There are other criteria being devised, but none of these has been universally satisfactory—we are still forced to rely on the teacher's judgment. We hope that eventually all educators will know about the hypermotor condition, will look for it, and will be able to communicate with the parents and the doctor. Once everyone realizes this is a treatable condition like any other, then something can be done about it.

This condition is diagnosed mainly from history, and there is almost no way (unless the child is extremely hypermotor) to recognize it in the doctor's office. However, I have had the experience of being able to differentiate between identical twins whose mother had trouble telling them apart. I have them sit on the examining table side by side and tell them not to move. From their behavior, I can sometimes tell which child was born first and which second. Usually, the second-born twin or the third-born in a set of triplets is more likely to have had oxygen deprivation. When the womb was contracting to deliver the first child, there could have been a lack of oxygen to the second child. This can lead to a slight hurt to the nervous system—just enough to impair concentration, decrease the attention span, and prevent the child from sitting completely still when asked to do so.

In something like 80 percent of hypermotor cases, medical authorities now feel there has been some such hurt to the victim's nervous system. There are many ways this can happen. The child might have suffered some lack of oxygen when the mother threatened to miscarry. The pregnant mother might have had a serious illness or infection that interfered with the supply of oxygen to the placenta. The baby might have been born by breech delivery, had the cord tightly around his neck, or it might have been necessary to take him by Caesarean section. The baby might have had a long hard delivery, or failed to revive or breathe right away. If the mother received anesthesia for painful labor contractions, this might have also anesthetized the child's

breathing reflexes. In the first few months of his life, he might
have had a collapsed lung, or have developed bronchitis, pneumonia, or whooping cough.

The proportion of adopted children with this syndrome is
higher than the usual (which is 4 percent of the general population). I can only relate this to the less-than-optimum ob-
stetrical care that is sought by the often indifferent, usually in-
experienced natural mothers.

There is also a remarkably high incidence of this condition
in prematurely-born children. Some authorities estimate that
something like half of all preemies have some slight nervous
system injury and are thus hypermotor. Children with other
neurological problems—such as congenital deafness or blindness
—often have a concomitant hypermotor condition. It also is seen
in children who have recovered from a rather severe neurological
disease, such as encephalitis after mumps, measles or chicken pox,
or meningitis. These children can be crippled to the extent of
being hypermotor without having any other real neurological
symptoms.

In fact, the hypermotor child usually does not display *any*
obvious neurological hurt. He may not be spastic or crippled,
and may not suffer from any loss of intelligence. He usually
seems bright, sharp, quick, eager, and anxious to learn, but because that part of his nervous system having to do with attention
span was once starved for oxygen, he is unable to focus attention
on any one thing for any length of time. We honestly do not
know precisely what anatomical area in the brain has suffered.
Autopsy investigations reveal no scar, cyst, or blood clot that
might pinpoint the damage. Someday, with better techniques, a
lesion or lesions may be discovered.

Some have asked why doctors have not noticed the hypermotor condition before. The problem has always been there, but
nobody was able to sit down and figure out the solution. Perhaps we were so busy with other problems of education that
these children were neglected. However, another explanation
may be that only in the last twenty years or so have we been
able to salvage prematures and other children suffering from
severe infections. Those who might have succumbed in the old
days to pneumonia, whooping cough, asthma, severe bronchitis,
or a collapsed lung are now being saved thanks to modern drugs.

However, their concurrent lack of oxygen has produced the hypermotor condition.

We have known for some twenty years that certain medicines prolong the attention span of these children, reduce some of their distractibility, and help them to stay in their seats. One such drug is amphetamine, sometimes known as Benzedrine. Another related drug is dextroamphetamine, sometimes known as Dexedrine. There are many forms of these drugs, and each has slightly different effects. The main thing these drugs do is to prolong the attention span. They allow a child to sit and think and do his work.

My wife is not very successful at sewing, so she does not like to sew. After she had just sewn a button on, someone would come back and say, "The button that you just sewed on fell off. Ha, ha! What's the matter?" My wife, who feels that she has enough things going the wrong way for her, decided to stop sewing. We have to get someone else to do it. However, she is a great cook. We have wonderful meals at our house. She is successful at this, so she keeps on cooking; the more successful she is, the more she cooks and the more she likes to do so. She gets positive feedback on the cooking and negative feedback on the sewing.

I think everybody is motivated by success in much the same way. If we are successful in something, we all keep trying and doing more of it, because we feel good about it. It is the same way with a child in school. The child who is doing well likes school because he is achieving and getting good comments from his teachers and parents. But the last child on the academic list knows he is the last one. His mother says, "I know you can do the work, if you just sit still and do it. Bring it home, and we'll help you." He is constantly being prodded and pushed into achieving his potential, but he gets so distracted in the classroom that he just cannot do it. He gets to hate school, because there is not much point in doing something every day when you are constantly being reminded that you are bad at it. I feel quite certain that if the condition is not controlled, then this child is a potential dropout.

It is fantastic how medicine can work. Within one hour or so, if the child is receiving the proper dose of the right medicine, his attention span stretches out. He will sit down and finish his work. He stops bothering the rest of the class. It may even improve his reading ability, and it certainly improves his concentration. The drug allows him to disregard unimportant stimuli, the little noises that are going on in every classroom.

With a child like this who may disturb the whole class, it is obvious that the teacher (who has a hard enough job teaching children when they are perfectly all right) needs to have something done so that she does not have to spend all her working hours with just him. She needs to be able to pay attention to the other children in the class.

Children do outgrow this condition, but often they are adolescents before this happens. Boys seem to be affected more often than girls.

So far as treatment is concerned, we have found that under age five it rarely works well, and that usually some less desirable side effects occur along with the beneficial ones. The most common drawback is loss of appetite. Most children who need a significant amount of medicine to control their hyperactivity fail to gain weight and sometimes will lose a pound or two. However, they can usually make up the loss during the summer vacation (most children don't need the medicine except on school days). My method has been to give the medicine every morning, Monday through Friday, but not to give it on Saturday and Sunday, and not through the summer.

The other side effect may be an inability to relax and go to sleep at night. The usual medicine, dextroamphetamine, is short-acting and starts to work in thirty to forty-five minutes. It is usually given at breakfast so that the beneficial effect has begun by the time the child is at school. It is usually assumed that after the first four to six hours, the medicine is pretty well out of the system (as is the case with most drugs). But many children whose bodies are poor at eliminating the medication carry some effects over for ten, twelve, or sometimes fourteen hours.

Accordingly, we may start a patient (depending on his size, of course) on half a tablet. The tablets are five milligrams; half a tablet would be two and a half milligrams. This would be the average dosage for a six-year-old, although he might need another half a tablet at noon. The child is probably getting his proper dose if the teacher notices improvement in his behavior. If there is no improvement, the dose should be progressively increased each day until the teacher is satisfied. An escalation of half a tablet each day is the best. Any side effects that may develop—such as mild appetite loss, slight insomnia, occasional headache, stomachache, crying, nervousness, or dilated pupils—usually disappear after a few days or weeks. The benefits of improved academic performance usually outweigh the disadvantages of those symptoms that do persist. If the side effects are really troublesome, or if there is no ultimate improvement in the classroom behavior, a different but related drug should be tried.

All children vary in the amount of medicine they can tolerate. I have had some patients who had to take four tablets in the morning and two more at noon. Because they were so uncontrollable at home, their mothers gave them another mild dose when they got home from school! I now have a patient who is so hypermotor at the age of twelve that he has to take eight tablets in the morning. His mother has found that if he takes only seven, he is up and out of his seat all the time at school and his grades are C's. If he takes eight tablets, he sits in his seat and gets A's. That last five milligrams is just enough to do the trick.

Because of its adverse effects on getting to sleep at night, the medicine is almost never given after five or six o'clock in the evening.

If dextroamphetamine does not prove beneficial (and the teacher and/or mother can tell in just a few days of juggling the dose), then careful doses of amphetamine (Benzedrine) should be tried. Sometimes this is ideal and sometimes it doesn't work, but again, use the same method—start with a small dose and build it up, while checking on its effects on sleep and appetite. Different combinations of the drugs may work; sometimes a tranquilizer has to be given along with the dextroamphetamine. Other types of amphetamines with different side chains may or may not prove beneficial, so most doctors get used to going down the list until they strike the proper one. If the child has this condition, one of these drugs will work—it is as easy as that.

Prior to the use of medication, it was common practice to retain these "immature" underachievers in the same grade. This usually served no useful purpose, and often bored the child and made him more disruptive.

If the academic year has been successful, the drug is best dropped for the summer. Each September the mother and the new teacher must reevaluate the child's behavior in the light of (1) the new teacher (some do better with these children than others), (2) passage of time (they do outgrow the need for medicine), and (3) the new class "personality" (seating arrangement, how many other hypermotor children, and so on). The new teacher should evaluate what he is doing in the first two weeks and report back to his mother *before September is out* whether or not he needs medicine. Some children develop insight as they get older and can feel what the pill does for them. They sense that somewhere deep inside them is the potential to sit still, and can make themselves do the work without medicine. But some "late bloomers" will need it all through high school.

I will be the last to say that purely psychogenic forces cannot cause this difficulty. Usually, however, psychological problems manifest themselves as withdrawal, fear, anxiety, or depression, and not as disorders of attention span or hyperactivity. Most "emotional" or "functional" symptoms result from the punitive, restrictive measures that teachers and parents have used to deal with the basic neurological fault.

Major traits of the hypermotor child are:

> Hyperactive behavior
> Short attention span
> Distractibility

The doctor or psychologist may see:

> Strephosymbolia (confusing *p* and *q*; *b* and *d*; reversing *was* and *saw*, *dog* and *god*)
> Dyslexia (specific reading disability out of proportion to intelligence)
> Visuo-sensory conceptual disorder related to the above
> Eye-hand coordination confusion
> Scatter of IQ test results between verbal (usually high) and performance (usually low)

The mother and/or the doctor may have observed:

> Hyperactivity in the womb
>
> Some oxygen deprivation before, at, or after delivery
>
> Premature, overdue, or postmature birth, smallness for age, or second of twins
>
> Whooping cough, pneumonia, or bronchitis requiring oxygen in the hospital
>
> Colic, fussy and demanding behavior, need to prop bottle
>
> Refusal to be cuddled, squirminess, ease of stimulation
>
> Sleep resistance (either light or restless sleeper)
>
> Tendency to be accident-prone, excessive climbing, falling, and swallowing poisons or adult medicines
>
> Constant asking of questions, and constant movement
>
> Inability to sit still even to eat or watch television without rocking or fiddling with something
>
> Eager, enthusiastic, and stimulating qualities that make the child nice to know but awful to live with

The teacher notices:

> Overactivity, frequent trips to bathroom or fountain, too much talking that is loud and out of turn, disruptive effect on class
>
> Restlessness, fidgeting, foot-tapping, annoyance of other children, inability to keep his hands to himself
>
> Knowledge and interest in everyone else's work, but failure to finish own
>
> Difficulty with arithmetic and spelling; failure in "self-control"
>
> Popularity and usually a lack of aggression or meanness, but overresponsiveness with laughing or crying
>
> Immaturity, daydreaming, underachieving

Drugs most commonly used:

> Dextroamphetamine sulfate (Dexedrine; Smith, Kline and French)
>
> Amphetamine sulfate (Benzedrine; Smith, Kline and French)
>
> Methylphenidate hydrochloride (Ritalin; Ciba)
>
> Methamphetamine hydrochloride (Desoxyn; Abbott)
>
> Deanolacetamidobenfoate (Deaner; Riker)

It is not unusual for mother, teacher, and doctor to discover a child is not only hypermotor, but also mean, stubborn, and impulsive. The impulsive, surly child will be described in the next chapter, but because both that child and the hypermotor one have been hurt by some sickness, the two conditions occasionally coexist. I have found that many hypermotor children have various additional behavior problems as a direct result of their failure in the classroom. They can become stubborn, obstinate, and uncooperative. Usually these symptoms disappear once they are on the proper medication and are having some academic success. But if their surly, stubborn behavior continues, then one certainly has to consider other psychiatric problems, or the possibility that other parts of the nervous system have been injured (as suggested in Chapter 6). It is not at all improbable that a child with this condition may have to be given not only dextroamphetamine, but also Dilantin or one of the tranquilizers.

I feel that I should reemphasize that putting a child on a drug is usually not the whole answer. In most cases, it solves the problem almost completely by breaking the cycle of failure and stopping the need for punitive control. The child, however, may need some psychiatric guidance and counseling from professional sources or at least from somebody outside the domestic scene. School counselors are a great help in redirecting his energies into socially acceptable channels.

I have mentioned that many of these drugs do not work properly on a child until the age of five or six. Still, that does not mean that they should not be tried. I would like to spend more time on the toddler who is a completely uncontrollable, highly charged, driven, impulse-ridden machine. Again, some hypermotor children do not display their distractibility until they are forced to sit still in the classroom. However, others are extremely hypermotor as soon as they start to get out of the crib. Once they are a year old and starting to get around the house, they are like spinning tops—knocking things over, pulling books off shelves, breaking windows, climbing up on the mantel, swinging from the chandelier, spilling everything in sight, falling into the toilet and out windows, jumping into the bathtub after filling the tub with scalding water—they seem to have no regard for personal safety.

Now, most toddlers act something like this, and a mother may need to have had a couple of normally rambunctious children before she can recognize when she is saddled with a real whirling dervish. Of course, the nursery school teacher can spot this child early and easily.

The mother usually has friends and neighbors who say such "helpful" things as, "If you weren't so nervous, your child wouldn't be so nervous." This is ridiculous—if she were not on edge and alert, her child would quickly hurt himself. She can only serve as a jailer who follows him around saving his life. Only the most patient mother can tolerate this role day after day without cracking up.

Some doctors are less than sympathetic with a mother who brings her driven child for help—the doctor, of course, is not living with him. You might try taking your child to a doctor who has had the same difficulty in his own home—he is usually more able to relate to the problem. Until recently, when we became more aware of the neurological implications, such children only served to antagonize us. They usually destroyed the examining room, and our patience along with it. Naturally, our first feeling was that the kid was not getting enough discipline, and we often suggested a good spanking. The mothers had of course tried several good spankings every hour with no success. They had found that natural mother love was turning, if not to hate, at least to strong dislike.

Medication is the only rational answer, but many seem to have adverse side effects on the under-five age group so they are worthless. In this situation, it is best to experiment with either Dilantin or one of the tranquilizers. Occasionally, some of the antihistamines are helpful. But most importantly, these children have to have an extremely structured environment, because the ordinary variations and stimuli in a home which most people can disregard are often too much for them. Everything has to be almost exactly the same day after day—meals served at the same time, bedtime at the same hour. Various activities have to be worked out so that the child knows what to expect from minute to minute.

I have noted that these children are more ticklish than most, and horseplay when father comes home in the evening over-excites them and makes relaxation for bedtime a major battle— they are all wound up again and cannot discharge their battery.

A family outing, a relative's visit, or a holiday, becomes bedlam, and all participants usually end up limp and weeping on the floor. Radios blaring, cars going by, visitors, door bells, and machines just serve as irritants; they should be minimized. You usually have to change the child's room into a padded cell. Otherwise, his impulses may destroy him if there are dangerous objects around.

A promising technique called *behavior modification* or *social engineering* has been found effective with some children with disruptive behavior. A child who acts this way usually gets negative responses from his mother by way of "no's," punishment, threats, and banishment. The mother is hard-pressed to find *any* favorable aspect of his daily life; to her, his rotten behavior seems continuous. But if offered some such minor reward as candy or money for sitting still or shutting up, he can later graduate to being rewarded simply by his mother's warm and positive response to his acceptable behavior. With practice, the vicious cycle can be broken.

Medicines often allow for a beginning. If they have been tried without success, they should be retried at least once a year in small doses that can be increased every few days. Time will make the nervous system more responsive to the medication. If children are this wild when they are toddlers, almost all will surely need treatment when they get to school.

References:
   Bradley, C., *Pediatrics*, vol. 5; pp. 24–37, 1950.
   Laufer and Denhoff; *Journal of Pediatrics*, vol. 50; pp. 463–474, 1957.

6 ◆◆◆◆◆

THE STUBBORN, SURLY CHILD

"If he weren't mine, I couldn't stand him."

Doctors of my generation who attended medical school during the 40's were excited because of the discovery of new, safe surgical techniques and many effective drugs. But our very first days of private practice revealed some big deficiencies in our medical education. Mothers, noting our eagerness to handle *all* their children's problems, handed us a few with less than classical symptoms. Many were of a psychiatric nature, and the gaps in our knowledge seemed to widen to an abyss.

The psychiatric courses we had in school were largely descriptive, and the psychoanalytic treatments were too involved. If something was not organic (structural or physical), then it had to be functional (emotional or psychiatric). However, it seemed odd that so many superficially normal women were producing children with such abnormal behavior. In many upset homes, we found the child's ornery behavior was predominantly responsible for the disruptive atmosphere.

Witness the case of Karen, age eight years, the third in a family of four girls. Karen's parents and their first two daughters had been living together in relative harmony, but a year or so

93

after Karen's birth, things changed for the worse. The mother felt Karen must have been suffering from the "third-child syndrome," whatever that is. She had treated all her children in the same way, fed them all the same milk, and loved them equally. All were in physically good condition. She was sure that unknowingly she must have done something to foul up Karen despite all her efforts to be fair. She called me in tears one day to say she could not stand her daughter another minute.

Actually, that mother was a happy, warm-hearted woman who did many wonderful things for her girls. They responded with warmth and cooperation—all except Karen, who did not seem to get the message. She always wanted 90 percent of what her mother could give, and left her sisters to split the last 10 percent. Karen turned a carefully planned picnic into a screaming, tearful shambles because she wanted to go to the beach instead of the mountains. Two weeks later, when the family acceded to her wishes by going to the beach, Karen had a temper tantrum because she wanted the mountains again! Everything had to go her way, and it was anybody's guess what that way would be.

Her mother could not remember if her freely admitted feelings about Karen had followed or preceded the ugly behavior. She did recall, though, that at fifteen months Karen had not ceased her tantrums after a reasonable length of time. Her physical and mental growth were now normal. She had no trouble in school. But her emotional responses seemed to have gotten stuck at the level of eighteen to twenty-four months. She was elbowing her way through life; she could not make friends. At home, she was stubborn, sullen, and uncooperative. She had difficulty "relating to her peers" in recess, in physical education classes, and in the cafeteria. Her moods were variable; her highs so high and her lows so low that she was unable to have any sort of meaningful relationships. The other children didn't know what to expect from her.

I had known this mother for a number of years, and felt that she had handled all her children in the proper way. So I looked back over Karen's chart to see whether there were any physical clues that might tip me off as to why she was acting so badly. Everything seemed normal. However, when she was a year old, she had contracted chickenpox from her eldest sister and had been quite sick at the time, running a high fever. (The second case of chickenpox in a family is often more severe than the first.) I then wondered if the fever had perhaps done some damage to her nervous system. I asked Karen's mother to take her for a brain-wave test—an electroencephalogram. The report came back that it was highly abnormal: Wave forms in the low range of three to ten per second were noted in all leads. (That is, the abnormality was happening all over her brain.)

At that time, we doctors felt the brain-wave test was as good as a chest X ray as a diagnosing tool. Because Karen's results were abnormal, I thought that her behavior was perhaps pre-epilepsy or sub-clinical epilepsy, and I put her on Dilantin, a medicine usually used to treat seizures. She was virtually a different child in about four days. Her mother could now admonish her without getting kicked. She could ask Karen to clean her room without incurring a violent rage.

Even if Karen had outgrown her abnormal brain waves, her unacceptable behavior might have continued and been termed "psychiatric." Age would have made her behavior problems increasingly difficult to treat. The nerves responsible for positive social reaction can degenerate if unused no matter how perfect the environment or therapy. In fact, her socially adequate responses might have been lost beyond recall by *any* medical or psychiatric treatment. If we had not done something to break her vicious cycle, I am convinced her rampages would have continued all her life.

Such children often blame others for their disagreeable actions. They carry a chip on their shoulder; they are defiant and stubborn. The world reacts to them correspondingly. As adolescents they will run away or become pregnant just to defy their parents. They lose their jobs because they fight with the boss, they break up their families because they treat little irritations as major ones. They continue to be explosive because they have learned to be.

Encouraged by the success of Karen's treatment, I began to use the same method with other mean children who came to the office. It was sometimes easy to identify the ones who would respond. If the mother was warm and friendly and one of her children was a "black sheep," medicine seemed to effect a dramatic change. Usually I could identify some episode in the early life of the child that might have hurt his nervous system.

Anoxia or oxygen deprivation seems to result in hyperactivity, short attention span and distractibility. (See Chapter 5). High fevers, dehydration, encephalitis and head injuries seem to be more common in the histories of children who have Karen's symptoms.

Jimmy's case was fairly clear-cut. He was the first born in a family of five children. His mother, somewhat nervous and insecure herself, was fortunately married to a rather stable man who helped her bear up under Jimmy's onslaught.

As he grew up, Jimmy pouted too much and was surly, stubborn, and uncooperative. He overreacted to the least little slight; his temper tantrums were too violent. The other children in the family certainly had their ups and downs, but they were friendly and cooperative. Because of the obvious contrast in behavior, his mother often wished she could have had Jimmy just as a "dry run" and disposed of him after she had learned something about child-rearing.

One day when Jimmy was eight, his mother woke at about five in the morning to find him turning and tossing in his bed and crying out. He was recovering from a convulsive seizure. His eyelids were flickering, his arms stiff. He was ashen, had broken out in a sweat, and had urinated. Because he had no fever to explain the spell and his blood calcium and sugar were normal, we took an EEG (electroencephalogram). The brain waves were abnormal, and he was placed on Dilantin to prevent further seizures. He is now pleasant and cheerful, cooperative, and easy to manage.

"Why didn't we put him on this medication before?" asked his mother. "He's a delight to have around. I love him now, but before, I must admit, I was getting to hate him." I told her I might have thought of the medication sooner if she had only told me how stubborn, mean, and aggressive he was.

"I was afraid you might think me a silly mother if I told you that," she said. "I was convinced his behavior was the result of my own mismanagement."

If Jimmy had been an only child, I would have been more likely to ascribe his problems to poor enviroment. But as in the case of Karen, it seemed more reasonable to blame the child for the disrupted home, inasmuch as the rest of the family seemed normal. In looking back, Jimmy had had a rather traumatic and extended labor and delivery, and this might—I say *might* —have slightly hurt his nervous system. Again, even had he outgrown his neurological difficulties (his tendency to epilepsy and aggressive behavior), he might eventually have developed a serious psychiatric problem.

It would be a neat, tidy, practical situation if we could run EEG's on all children with behavior abnormalities, verify the diagnosis, and put them on medicine. The trouble with this approach is that it does not always work, for several reasons: (1) Parents may refuse to admit that a problem exists. (2) The EEG has been found to be not as reliable as we used to think. (3) Medicines don't always work on everyone.

But the success rate is high enough. Certainly unacceptable behavior *can* be the direct result of parental attitudes. But a child who is sullen, stubborn, and impulsive may just as easily cause his parents to react in the same key. Once the pattern is established, parent and child respond to each other negatively as soon as they get in the same room. If it is so degrading, enervating, and unpleasant, why don't the participants stop? They can't. It is locked in, like a knee-jerk reflex or an itchy hive.

Some parents can pinpoint the inciting event, such as Karen's sickness or Jimmy's difficult delivery. Most families, however, drift into turmoil so slowly and unobstrusively that they are unaware of what is happening—until friends, relatives, or teachers point out the deviation. Most hope it is a phase that will pass. Many mothers believe they are responsible for the sickness in their family. Like fighting quicksand, however, they sink deeper. They need strong rescue techniques.

Typical home situations fall into four categories:
(1) The reasonably normal children of fairly normal parents account for most of our patients and for about 75 percent of the population. Any problems in this first group should be temporary and can be solved with reassurance, education, reorientation, and insight.
(2) About 10 to 15 percent of children have some neurological hurt. When one of these children tries to relate to his normal mother, he misinterprets or garbles her messages. When he overreacts, his mother then gets a distorted message from *him*. Faced with an unnatural reaction, she responds ineffectively with

frustration and anxiety—and a negative reflex pattern is begun, as with Karen and Jimmy.

Group (2) has problems that require social and educational engineering, drugs, and possibly psychological help. If the Gordian knot is untangled in time, the psychiatrist may not be needed. If medicine improves a child's mood and response patterns, his normal family will be able to alter their inappropriate reactions. The child can be rewarded for socially acceptable behavior, which hopefully will continue after the medicine is stopped.

(3) When a normal child gets little love, encouragement, or positive rewards from a cold, rejecting, or punitive set of parents, he may quit his normal progress toward maturity and become fixed at some infantile level of social response.

(4) A neurologically damaged or genetically unbalanced child born into a neurotic home has almost no chance. He will most likely end up battered physically and emotionally.

These latter two groups must account for 5 to 10 percent of all families. Pediatricians rarely see these often unwanted children simply because their parents don't care. However, their behavior becomes obvious to the police during adolescence. By the time their deviant behavior begins to really become harmful, their fixed patterns make treatment long, difficult, or impossible.

This may be the reason why specialists dispute each other's jurisdiction over behavior problems. The pediatrician, who sees many problems in normal families, would suspect organic or neurological causes. The psychiatrist, who sees neurotic parents with deviant children, would conclude that most abnormal behavior is environmentally produced. But in reality, these two explanations blend into one another. Somewhere deep in the brain's intertwining circuits, neurology and psychiatry are intimately interconnected.

Brain research is a new field. Until recently, we knew only those areas that controlled muscle use and received sensory stimuli. The brain was supposed to be only a switchboard, moving appropriate muscles in response to the various messages it received from the body. Now, clever experiments in animals have indicated that deeper, minute brain centers are able to control rage, fear, laughter, sexual excitement, and even hunger and sleep. Some neurosurgeons have removed corresponding areas of the brain to correct incapacitating behavior or seizure problems. Medical schools find it easier to teach neurology and psychiatry as separate subjects, but the brain itself does not seem to be aware of this academic dichotomy. Since our knowledge of the brain's inaccessible areas is still inadequate, we cannot rule out structural, biochemical, or electrical anomalies as factors of "emotional" disease. Why have we not developed a neuro-psychiatric theory that would encompass all mental problems? A malfunctioning nerve in the thalamus could affect the brain as much as a cruel father. Diabetes is controllable with insulin. Will an unknown chemical control the as-yet-undetected bio-chemical imbalance or enzyme lack causing some psychoses, such as schizophrenia?

At the present stage of knowledge, theories of behavior problems are not as useful as early identification and treatments. You are the chief historian of your child, and your description is usually all we have to go on. Here are some clues to neurological problems:

He overresponds to slight physical or emotional trauma.

He is impulse-ridden.

He acts out his aggression.

He has no control over his emotions.

He laughs and cries too easily.

A three- or four-year-old has violent temper tantrums like the fifteen- to eighteen-month-old child.

He hurts animals or wrecks toys.

After a wild outburst he says to his mother, "I'm sorry, Mother. I love you very much." "Well," says the mother, "let's try not to do *that* again." Then in five or ten minutes, he does it again. He is a Jekyll and Hyde, the black sheep of the family.

He elbows his way through life. He is a bully, he has to win every game he plays. He has to be able to ride his bike the first time he gets on it, or there is something wrong with the bike.

He has no friends, or the friends he has are invariably younger than he.

He is never invited to other homes for a birthday party or to stay overnight.

When they choose up sides to play games in school, he is the last one chosen. Classmates call him "klutz," "wimp," and "kook."

Such children often get into fights. Their attitude is one of stubborn hostility. They seem to pout more and be depressed and unhappy. When asked about their behavior, they always have a reason—it was someone else's fault. They operate on impulse: "Here's a rock; there's a window. Let's throw the rock through the window." "There's an old man. Let's call him names."

As they get older, their behavior becomes more antisocial. In adolescence, they may be the ones most likely to steal something just because it is available.

"There are the keys in the ignition; let's steal this car." They drive away, run out of gas, and the police catch them.

"Why did you do that?"

"I don't know. I just had to do it."

These children *may* do well in schoolwork, but they have trouble at lunch, in physical education, or after school. After a while, they get a reputation for being troublemakers. No matter what happens in the classroom, they are blamed (and usually it is justified). They're more likely to be truants from school, blaming some real or imagined pressure. Their report cards will consistently show "poor citizenship." They may or may not have a short attention span and be distractible. They may or may not be hypermotor or hyperactive.

A child's social adaptability in school is the real test of his ability to "relate." It is also a good forecast of his social potential as an adult (hence, the importance of nursery school). With twenty or thirty like-aged children, it is usually easy to spot the sick, the hyperactive, and the bully. The teacher recognizes the one who stands in the corner, is stubborn and defiant, kicks the chair or just sits on the floor, has a temper tantrum, stamps his feet, or makes noise.

Armed with a mother's story and a teacher's evaluation, we are frequently not surprised to find confirmation in our own notes. Child's reaction in our office: he cried for fifteen or twenty minutes after a DPT immunization shot, where the average child only whimpers for a minute or two. He over-reacted to the examination when he was a year old. He was extremely fearful at two or three when most children can be jollied out of their anxiety. I found examples of overreaaction in Karen's chart after her bout with chickenpox: "18 months— screamed," "2 years—really fought," "3 years—kicked, pouted, couldn't be undressed," "4 years—jerked stethoscope out of my ears."

The psychologist is often consulted when the mother, the teacher, and the doctor need diagnostic confirmation. He can frequently attest to the presence of neurological injuries, estimate intelligence, and determine the part played by environmental and emotional factors.

I have mentioned the use of the brain-wave test, the electro-encephalogram, as a possible way of diagnosing children with strong aggressive responses. However, documented studies now indicate that no high correlation exists between bad behavior and abnormal brain waves. The test largely measures surface electrical potential difference; underneath all sorts of violent things may be going on that escape this otherwise sensitive machine. Many children have normal brain waves and obvious neurological damage. Others have very abnormal brain waves and perfectly normal behavior. A borderline EEG can be read as normal by one neurologist and abnormal by another. Therefore, most of us have abandoned the EEG as a sure-fire diagnostic aid in behavior problems.

After a problem child has been identified by the mother (who can't stand him), the nursery school teacher (who can't take him another day), the psychologist (who scores his abnormal responses), and the pediatrician (who got kicked), then some treatment has to be organized. However, it is naive to reorganize only the child's attitudes and then put him back into the same atmosphere—he will quickly revert to his familiar response pattern. He must feel he is winning or is successful when he behaves in a socially acceptable way. Thus, authorities agree that one has to change the whole domestic scene in order to achieve any degree of success.

Behavior responses result from a complicated, interconnecting series of nerve signals. If a finger relays the word that the stove is hot, the normal brain stores the fact away as valuable knowledge. If a child's loving mother indicates joy and approval when he takes his first step, his brain stores up the approval; he'll take more steps. A child with straight legs often discovers he can run fast. The more he runs, the better he runs. The better he runs, the more he is complimented and encouraged to run.

Success breeds success, and failure invites failure. A child with a neurological hurt may be unable to succeed at some simple task. If his or his mother's standards are too high for his personal development level, he becomes frustrated by "negative feedback" and becomes angry, hostile, or sullen, depressed and withdrawn. He expects to fail and to be chewed out for it. Each time he finds himself in a similar situation, he reacts in the same immature way. It becomes a habit; a reflex that the child and environment have created between them.

The more a nervous-system pathway is utilized, the more readily it is used again. Conversely, *unused* nerve pathways actually degenerate and become unresponsive to stimuli. For instance, if a child has crossed eyes, his brain compensates by suppressing the image it receives from one eye. If not forced to function, the eye soon becomes blind permanently; the nerves are structurally present but unable to carry messages to the visual area of the brain. (A deaf baby babbles at first, but he soon becomes mute or talks nonsense because he does not hear any rewarding sounds from his mother.) He often becomes hostile when his environment doesn't answer him in a way he is able to understand.

Whether classical Freudian theories or more pragmatic approaches are used, basic therapy is the same: You must break the vicious cycle, stop negative feedback, and unlearn the old, bad response patterns. Seize on the child's socially *acceptable* responses and reward them. The earlier the age, the easier.

Almost no family has enough insight to be able to solve its own disruptive problems without outside help. Most pediatricians do not feel equipped or confident enough to handle the neurotic mother whose unconscious feelings are thwarting her child's progress toward maturity. (However, it is amazing how normal some children can be in their unbalanced homes; the urge to grow and mature is very strong.) Doctors are more likely to try medicines and short-term family engineering on the disturbed child. Perhaps if he feels and acts better, his mother can relax and discard the attitudes she adopted when he first began to irritate her. If she is normal, perhaps she can then reward him with love and praise. Because both child and environment (mother) are changed, perhaps each will continue to reinforce the other. New, hitherto unused healthy nerve responses can be put to use—once the vicious cycle is broken.

The technique of *behavior modification* as mentioned in Chapter 5 is helpful in reversing unacceptable behavior. First, a mother must understand how she is perpetuating her child's poor responses. She then gives him some appropriate reward (a toy, piece of candy, or lavish praise) for some ever-so-slight but definitely *positive* social response. (Examples: he did not throw food on the floor, brought a friend home, smiled for one second, or lost a game without a temper tantrum.) Instead of punishing him for the transgressions that seem to occupy 99 percent of his day, she showers him with love for the hard-to-notice one percent. In a few weeks, his "good" time may be up to 55 percent and his "bad" down to 45 percent. He's better because she's better because he's better, and so on.

Medication may enhance the improvement rate especially when the parents are normal and concerned. Dilantin has been mentioned; rare and temporary but dangerous side effects make its use somewhat risky. Barbiturates usually dope a child or make him wild. Phenidate, amphetamines, imipramine, compazine, and benadryl all have their uses.

But even with drugs, we can do little unless the mother is mature and confident in her role. She is most often considered the villain or hero because she is most often part of her child's behavior arc. After all, she is a product of her own early experiences. If her childhood was fairly normal, she will respond properly to her own child's maturation.

No other two people react and communicate like a mother and her child. Your mind must be free of marital, financial, health, and in-law problems so you can feed warmth, security, and love into your baby's psyche. I am really impressed by the hope and endurance of a mother despite the frequent sabotage by a selfish husband, critical relatives, and a basically nasty child. The real trick in child-rearing is to balance your discipline, punishment, and "no's" with enough love and acceptance of natural gregariousness to allow your child to feel he is a worthwhile member of the family. We all need to feel that somebody else cares—that somebody is listening.

I am in no way advocating that you rear a generation of squares—perfectly behaving, obedient sheep who never question the dictates of their older generation. I would just like to see our children grow up socially aware, achieving their goals and fulfilling their potentials without hurting others. If your two-year-old repeatedly hits another child to get a toy, you would scold him and he would understand that he had gone too far. He would then file that information in his memory. If his nerve synapses are functioning, he would show more control in the next similar situation; and so on until adult maturity. If your seven-year-old did the same thing, then he either did not learn impulse control from you or he *could* not because of a defective nervous system.

You can sense what sort of a child you have by the time he is twelve to eighteen months old.

Normal: he smiles easily, responds to cuddling, enjoys play-time, is upset but not violent at separation, makes up to people, is refreshed after sleep and satisfied after eating, laughs and smiles more than he cries and frowns, and seems remorseful after scolding or discipline—at least for a while.

Abnormal: he acts younger than his chronological age, cries easily, becomes sick when crying, cries because he is crying, cannot be "jollied" out of a bad mood, overreacts to tickling, is excessively shy or distant with strangers, is always afraid, "attacks" food and toys as if they are enemies, reacts with violence to normal discipline, and has a defiant, chip-on-the-shoulder attitude.

The world has enough violence. Medical science has yet to devise a technique or machine to diagnose children prone to perpetuate it. Schools, churches, and governments do what they can to channel anger and hostility into athletic prowess or heated discussion. We need cheerful, intelligent mothers to rear the next generation, and we cannot let any child scuttle their efforts.

FOUR CATEGORIES OF SICK CHILDREN

	Hyperactive	Surly, mean	Fearful, timid	Compulsive, neat
	Short attention span Distractible Talkative Underachiever Immature Restless Accident-prone	Fights, no friends Has to win, rages Breaks toys Projects blame Acts out Aggressive Lights fires Temper outbursts	Clinging, anxious Tearful Cannot face new situations Clumsy, loner Depressed, withdrawn No friends Tired, sickly	Tries too hard Must be top of class Tense, tics, twitches Ulcer prone, stays up late Migraine headaches Nervous stomach
Causes	Oxygen lack Prematurity	High fever Convulsions	Pregnancy late in life Intrauterine factors	Genetic
Contributing Factors	No limits Permissive environment	No love Punitive parents Constant devaluation Genetic	No love Devaluation	Demands for achievement Rigid home
Treatment	Amphetamine Methylphenidate Social engineering	Phenobarbital Imipramine Dilantin Psychotherapy	Imipramine Dilantin Behavior modification	Lower goals Less pressure Tranquilizers Psychotherapy

7 ◆◆◆◆◆

ALLERGIES

"Maybe he's allergic to me."

I am amazed at how often an allergy can bypass the usual obvious symptoms of sneezing and watery eyes and mask itself as a psychological difficulty. One of my three-year-old patients showed me how an allergy can appear, at least superficially, as a psychosomatic problem. In this particular case, Frank, a child of divorced parents, was living with his mother. Frank went right off to sleep at seven o'clock at night, but he'd wake up every twenty minutes with some excuse such as only a three-year-old can concoct. He'd need a drink of water, so his mother would get him one. In a minute or so he'd be back to sleep for another twenty minutes; then he'd wake up again and say he had to brush his teeth because he had forgotten. So he would brush his teeth and go back to sleep for another twenty minutes. Then he would be up to urinate, because of the water he drank forty minutes before. In another twenty minutes, he'd be hungry (I suppose he worked up an appetite by getting out of bed so often).

This routine usually went on until about two o'clock in the morning, when he would go to sleep once and for all until seven.

His mother had tried discipline, scoldings, spankings; she had even taken to getting in bed with him to make him feel secure. She was a normal person and needed six to eight hours of sleep herself. But as you and I know, once we adults are awakened, it takes us about fifteen or twenty minutes to relax and go back to sleep. The mother would sleep for a minute or two and be up twenty, and her boy would sleep for twenty and be up for a minute or two. *He* felt fine the next day, but she was exhausted. She had taken Frank to a doctor who treated him for worms, because as a rule anyone who wakes up at night should be treated for worms. The doctor had also found and taken care of a little ear infection, but Frank was still up every twenty minutes. He then suggested some phenobarbital to help get Frank in the habit of sleeping through the night, but it only made him dopey. He awakened as usual, and staggered around and bumped into things.

Immediately one thinks, "Aha! Anything that goes wrong here must be the result of this broken home." I'm not going to defend divorce, but I have the feeling that every once in a while a broken home is better than one filled with hate and bickering. Frank's doctor had no other suggestions and thought, "Well, his nighttime wakefulness must be caused by the insecurity of his broken home. He's waking up because he needs reassurance that his mother isn't going to leave him like his father did."

His mother felt guilty and inadequate for being away from Frank so much. "Well," she thought, "I guess there's no other answer. I'm gone all day, and he wakes up at night—therefore, he must be insecure. I'd better quit my job and stay home with him. If that doesn't work, I'll go to a child guidance clinic or a psychiatrist for help. If that doesn't work, maybe I'll board him out."

She spoke to me about her rash decision. I could find nothing wrong with her son. Of course, it is difficult to diagnose anxiety and insecurity by the routine physical examination. We get a few clues if the three-year-old hides behind his mother, screaming, "No! No! Go home; go home!" But not Frank; he stood in the middle of the room clad only in the dubious security of underwear and socks, smiled, looked in my eyes, shook hands and said, "Hi." He did not appear anxious to me.

If a patient has stomachaches or headaches without physical or emotional cause, or if his symptoms do not fit a classical dis ease pattern, then we think of an allergy. So I asked the mother about allergies.

"Oh, yes." she said, "When he was a small baby, he used to throw up his cod-liver oil."

"Aha!" I said. "Maybe that's it. Why don't you cut out the cod-liver oil?"

"He hasn't had any for a long time," she replied.

That obviously wrecked the cod-liver oil theory. She also denied any sort of nose picking, asthma, eczema, hives, or any other peculiar rashes that could be remotely connected to an allergy. I even asked about changes in bowel habits or gas, but she said there was really nothing at all in that department. Then I asked her about vitamins.

She was not sure how good a diet Frank was getting from his daytime baby-sitter, so she thought it smart to supplement his diet with Brand X vitamins. She was too busy and tired in the morning to worry about vitamins, so she gave them to Frank at suppertime, in the evening after she got home.

"Aha!" I said. "Maybe that's it."

"Hah!" she said. "It couldn't make that much difference." But that night she did not give him his vitamins. Frank did not wake up. He slept right through the night, and his mother got a good night's sleep for the first time in about eight months. (She almost lost her job because she relied on Frank to wake her up in the morning.) The next night she again withheld his vitamins and purposely sat up to see what would happen. He slept through the second night in a row. This happened the third and fourth nights. The fifth night, as a test, she gave him his vitamins as usual—and sure enough, he woke up every twenty minutes.

This boy had outgrown his cod-liver oil allergy, at least to the extent that it didn't make him throw up. But perhaps there was just enough cod-liver oil in Brand X vitamins to make his intestines develop a cramp every twenty minutes. This cramp was not so terrific that he would double up and roll on the floor. His mother had no way of knowing it was his stomach that was bothering him; it was just enough pain to wake him up. Feeling uncomfortable, he would provide some silly excuse to be up and around. He'd go back to sleep, but twenty minutes later the vitamins would go around another corner in his intestines and give him another little cramp. At two or three in the morning, when

the vitamins were sufficiently absorbed or digested, the cramps
would stop and he would sleep. Then he would be all right until
the next evening when he got another dose. What appeared to
be an obvious psychological problem was traced, by some detective work, to an allergy.

I have often thought what might have happened if this boy
had been taken out of his broken home and put in a better structured one—a home where the mother always remembers to give
vitamins in the morning; always remembers to salt the oatmeal;
always remembers to kiss her husband good-bye when he leaves
for work. With such a perfect wife and mother, of course, this
child would get his vitamins in the morning, and in the excitement of play during the day he wouldn't notice these minor
stomachaches. Naturally he wouldn't wake up in the night because the vitamins would have been digested by bedtime. Everyone would have naturally assumed that the "broken-home syndrome" had been the real culprit after all.

Fortunately, we solved this particular problem. I am not saying
that Frank will be a *perfectly* normal adult; maybe his broken
home is going to foul up his psyche some way. But I think he has
enough strength of character and his mother enough intelligence
and sense of humor that she can rear him properly. It would have
been silly to go to all the trouble of relocating the poor child
just because he was allergic to vitamins.

Looking back on this case, the solution seems ridiculously
simple, but at the time it appeared profoundly complex, for a
variety of reasons. Our medical school training on allergies dwelt
mainly on classical manifestations: asthma, eczema, and hay
fever. We were unprepared for the other infrequently recognized symptoms of an allergy. By the time the sensitive patient
arrived in our office, *he* usually had made the diagnosis and only
wanted relief. We had also learned that if there is nothing physical to be found behind a symptom, we must diagnose a neurotic
or at least a psychosomatic condition. But the really disturbing
feature we did not realize about allergies is how common they
really are.

The child with a typical allergy usually feels irritable—because
of the inherent nature of his reaction, the medicine used to treat
it, or the lack of sleep resulting from the symptoms. The mother
usually makes allowances for his poor disposition because she

knows the reasons for it. But if he is suffering from headaches, gas, diarrhea, constipation, sluggishness, earaches, cough, frequent urination, stomachaches, or meanness, the doctor is often baffled because the organs in question are perfectly healthy. The mother can only assume that *she* is causing the symptoms, and reacts by ignoring or overreacting to them—thus initiating a pattern that can lead to hypochondria in the child. She may also become hostile and punitive, on the logical assumption that the kid is going out of his way to be a nuisance and miss school.

If parents were more aware of the tremendous variety of symptoms that allergies can produce, they could use a little detective work to solve many sticky problems. If Frank's mother had said, "Every time he gets vitamins for supper, he awakens every twenty minutes during the night," I would have seen the connection and responded with, "Sounds like an allergy; why don't you give the vitamins in the morning, stop them, or change brands?" Elementary! Before you label your child as a malingerer or neurotic, try some elimination tests. It usually takes only about two to four days to be sure, so you will not have lost much valuable time if it is really something else.

Food allergies will manifest themselves in a variety of ways. I once read an article written by a doctor of internal medicine who was trying to help explain the nature of headaches. He categorized them according to frequency, location, type, and mode of onset; and whether they were due to pressure, tension, pulled muscles, blood-vessel inflammations, or pinched nerves. On this list of headaches was the one-sided type, a vascular headache as distinct from migraine. This pounding, throbbing headache seems to be right in one blood vessel and can be temporarily relieved by holding the vessel flat. It seems to be relieved by caffeine and aspirin. This doctor went so far as to say that 40 percent of these headaches are due to allergies, and I have since come to believe his percentage is fairly accurate.

Allergy headaches are usually one-sided, but may be all over. They appear two to twelve hours after the offending food is consumed and may last for a day or two. Chocolate, milk, corn, wheat, eggs, nuts, fish, vitamins, drugs, citrus fruits, and tomatoes are the usual offenders. Some children (and adults) feel tired and develop pallor and dark circles under the eyes. Others become anxious or nervous and have cold sweats. A rare child will abandon play or withdraw from toys or friends, as if depressed. A few change into hostile, mean, snarly animals. I know a man who has a needling, tense, bitchy wife; his headaches disappeared when he ran out of chocolate to stir in his milk. He *should* have headaches without the chocolate, but he doesn't. Recently, a ten-year-old boy was thought to have a brain tumor until the offending milk was discontinued.

Stomachaches from food sensitivities may be noticed only as a vague sense of fullness; few are so violent as to make one suspect an abdominal emergency. They may or may not be associated with gas, diarrhea, vomiting, or constipation. Most always, the distress is at or around the navel. A child with a minor stomachache may find it convenient to magnify the problem if doing so serves some purpose such as keeping him home from school. Such a condition may start as an allergy but become psychosomatic.

Urinary symptoms are most often associated with fluid components of the diet—milk, citrus and tomato juice, and chocolate. Other fruits may be responsible, but in general the liquid things seem to bother a patient's bladder more than solid ones. Urgency and frequency of urination—as if the bladder were too small and sneezing—are usual symptoms. About one of twenty bed-wetters is cured by eliminating the above offenders.

I was once amazed to read an article by someone who professed to be a bed-wetting expert. Again, he found that 40 percent (!) of *his* patients' bed-wetting was due to an allergy.

Some patients develop an irritation or swelling at the base of the bladder or in the first part of the urethra, which precludes emptying the bladder completely. A secondary infection, like a sinus infection, then develops. The penis or vagina may itch, and the socially indifferent child may rub the area constantly, to the embarrassment of parents who misinterpret the activity as masturbation or some "oversexed" condition.

Nasal symptoms that sound as if the adenoids were enlarged are most frequently caused by a milk allergy that stimulates mucous glands to pour out their tenacious secretions. The victim constantly clears his throat, snorts, and produces very disagreeable snoring sounds in an effort to dislodge this rubbery phlegm from his palate. He often feels as if his ears are plugged, and manipulates his jaw in an irritating, futile effort to open up his Eustachian tubes.

Aching joints, muscle pains, canker sores, pustules, boils, acne, laryngitis, abnormal tongue sensations, mysterious swellings about the body, anal fissures, and itches can be distantly connected with food and inhalation sensitivities.

I have mentioned the frequency of allergies in babies. Our first contact with an allergic child usually occurs in the first month of his life when he develops one or all of several problems: loose, green, gassy stools; much distress or cramping; vomiting (more than just spitting up); and terrible weepy, raw skin rashes on his cheeks, spreading down to his neck or behind his ears, on the front part of his elbows, or behind his knees. This is usually due to milk allergy. Some children also develop phlegm or a gurgly noise as if they had a dripping faucet in the throat; others actually develop asthma. An allergy usually takes a few days or weeks to develop because the tissues or "shock organs" require a few exposures before they become sensitive. About one baby in twenty will become allergic to cow's milk, and about half of these continue to have allergic problems all their lives. In upwards of 60 percent of these babies, there is an allergic background in the family.

The following has happened in the office: I will be treating a three-month-old baby, say, for an obvious milk allergy. One day, when his mother brings him in she brings her husband along, too, just to show him what a pediatrician looks like. As we are talking, I am suddenly amazed at how this baby is the image of his father; same color hair and eyes, same little dimple in the chin, same general body build. I cannot help but ask the father if he has a milk allergy, too. Of course he denies it. "I have a nervous stomach," he says. "The doctor's taken X rays and found an irritable duodenum, but that's all he can find. I'm sure it's business pressure. The boss is on my back all the time; my wife is screaming at me at home; the kids are hollering, and the baby's milk costs three or four times what the regular formula would. I just know that's what brings on my stomach distress and burping and gas attacks."

"Well," I say, "that certainly may be true, but why don't you quit milk for a while and see what happens?"

"No," he replies, "my doctor suggested I drink milk because if this is a pre-ulcer condition, the milk is the best thing for it."

"Well," I suggest, "there are some other things you can take that act as antacids. Why don't you see what no milk will do?"

His answer is, "But I *know* it's psychosomatic—when the company sends me to a convention in Las Vegas, I don't have any stomach trouble at all. When I'm out of the office and away from the pressures at home, it all goes away."

Of course, I have to suppress the suggestion that people at conventions in Las Vegas don't drink much milk, and could it be he is not allergic to whiskey? I wonder how often an executive flaunts any bodily complaint that implies that he is working at peak capacity. If he seems to have some neurotic symptoms, he likes to display it because it is a status symbol—he is a hard worker in the mainstream of competitive American business. Nevertheless, if you or your husband have a history of specific allergies, they should be your prime suspects in any investigation of your child's problems.

The nonworking, blissfully unpressured baby usually outgrows his milk sensitivity by the time he is twelve to eighteen months old. His mother is greatly relieved to find he can drink milk safely, except of course, it is now time for her to start cutting *down* on his milk consumption! It is also time for upwards of 40 percent of the babies who had milk allergies to develop inhalation allergies. This variability of allergic manifestations, their tendency to move from one system to another, behooves any mother to make plans for the future.

We suggest that reasonable efforts be made to minimize the more common sensitizing foods, inhalants, and contactants. This is partly why most doctors recommend a slow introduction to solid foods, especially to such foods as citrus fruits, tomatoes, eggs, wheat, pork, nuts, and green vegetables. These are most likely to produce allergic responses, and should be introduced only after the child is one year old. Meanwhile, you should also keep the child's room free of dust.

These things are routine. Most children can compensate for a few allergies; don't push another one on them. If they are eating foods to which they are sensitive and breathing dust—and then the weather changes, or there is some emotional excitement, or a nice dander-filled cat or dog comes by—then, wham! The combination can trigger a bad attack that may take some time and expense to correct.

Some have compared the allergic patient to a bathtub into

which streams of water are flowing from a number of spigots (the allergic irritants). Most sensitive people have several spigots running. If the ouflow drain is big enough, he has no symptoms. But if the spigots are all running full blast, he will soon overflow with asthma, eczema, hay fever, and other reactions. You can turn off a few spigots by getting rid of dogs, rugs, milk, feathers, and emotional problems—or else have your doctor open up the drain with desensitizing shots or anti-allergy medicines.

Another common allergy manifests itself between six and eighteen months. The baby develops an inordinate number of colds. Let me define the term *cold:* It is a virus-caused respiratory infection manifested by a watery, runny nose, and usually bleary, red-rimmed eyes. In the first day there is some sneezing and a slight cough due to the drippage down the throat. A baby up to two years of age sometimes runs a fever of 100° to 102° F. for twenty-four to forty-eight hours. The watery, drippy nose goes on for seven days. If the discharge from the nose turns purulent —green or yellow—it means a secondary bacterial infection has taken over. This is not serious in itself, but occasionally progresses to a throat, ear, eye, sinus, bronchial, or skin infection that demands treatment with sulfa, penicillin, or some appropriate antibiotic.

In the first few years of life, the drippy nose seems to be normal, just as a child who messes with his food or wets his pants is considered normal up to a certain age. In an attempt to establish just what "normal" is, doctors and epidemiologists have made statistical studies of how many colds children have from the age of one to six. The nationwide average is somewhere between six and eight respiratory infections per child per year. This seems a fantastic number, but it appears to correlate with what we find in practice; about every month and a half, a child comes down with a cold or runny nose.

Allergic children are apparently even more susceptible. The child in question may or may not have had any previous history of milk or inhalant allergies, and there may be no known family tendency. Many parents believe that if they eat properly, take vitamins, and get their rest, they will avoid "colds." They see the "snotty-nosed" children of their friends and vow *they* won't *ever* have children like that. Thus, many mothers bring their children to the office because they can't stand their own child's

drippy nose for one more minute, but most of the time we cannot find anything really wrong with him. He may have circles
under his eyes, he may look a little pale, but he is not anemic.
He is on a fairly good diet; he may even be taking some extra
vitamins. His lungs are clear, his tonsils not too big, and his ear
drums perfectly normal, but he continues to have a green or yellow pus-filled nose.

I have tried, as most doctors have, to do something—perhaps
putting the child on an antibiotic or sulfa drug. Within two or
three days the condition clears up. But as soon as the medicine
stops or he gets a new cold, the green or yellow purulent discharge recurs. There is controversy among the allergists as to
whether there is such a thing as "an allergy to your own bacteria" or "an allergy to yourself." If every time a child gets a
cold he then develops a secondary, purulent rhinitis along with
asthma or spastic bronchitis (during which he has to work to
exhale), this implies that he is allergic to his own bacteria.

Even with the run-of-the-mill runny nose, it seems helpful
to give these children three or four dead bacteria shots. (The
bacteria vaccine is made from the victim's own nasal discharge or
a stock solution of six or seven of the usual bacteria found in
most peoples' noses and throats. These killed bacteria are injected into the sufferer in an attempt to "immunize" or "desensi-
tize" him against the bacteria.) Success with this method has
been upwards of 70 to 80 percent. Some patients need to have a
booster shot occasionally when the condition recurs. In any case,
the treatment improves the condition by reducing the number
of secondary nose, ear, and bronchitis infections, and the need
for expensive antibiotics.

If allergies can be controlled, the child will have fewer colds
and will be less susceptible to bronchitis and croup. Asthmatic
bronchitis attacks are often accompanied by high fevers, convulsions, and cyanosis, which could conceivably hurt the developing nervous system. One common secondary infection is
otitis media or middle-ear infection. Even if adenoids and tonsils
are removed to halt the ear infections, the operation still may not
solve the riddle because the initial allergy is still operative. The
tonsils and adenoids may act as sponges and soak up the material
flowing over them, so I would assume that eliminating this drain-

age might serve to protect these islands of lymph tissue from infection. Most children withstand these infections, but if they seem really beset with colds and sniffles, allergies should be suspected. A doctor may not be aware of the frequency of his patients' colds, so the mother may have to document the number for him. Incidentally, anemic children have about double the "cold rate" of the nonanemic.

I must admit I have no way of knowing whether any one child will outgrow this irritating condition. I have made no controlled studies with identically snotty-nosed twins, in which one was treated and the other was not. The individuals I have treated all had this purulent discharge until they got the shots, and then it usually lessened or disappeared.

When an allergy is at fault, sometimes an alert mother will put the picture together so nicely that the diagnosis is easy.

"At eight months of age, I changed from formula to whole milk, and he's been cranky ever since." (Whole milk has not been processed as much as evaporated or prepared milk and thus is more allergenic.)

"We moved to an old house and he has had a cough and cold every three weeks." (Housedust, mold in walls, new bedding, etc.)

"We got rid of our cat, but John still sneezes and wheezes." (The cat's dander is still in the furniture.)

Some children have little visible discharge out of the front of the nose, but make a terrible snorting, sniffing sound as if a bunch of rubber bands were dangling down the back of the nose and throat. Sometimes the dead bacteria shots will control this also, but the child's nasal discharge has to be green or yellow, and the other forms of inhalation allergy have to be ruled out.

The shots will *not* work if the child has a *clear*, watery, runny nose and if he is sneezing and picking his nose a great deal. This implies that his major problem is due to inhalants. Some attention must be given to food and bacteria, but environmental control is essential if you would relieve the sniffing, rubbing, picking, fiddling, worrying, and wiping that goes on about the nose.

Sometimes, just eliminating dust from the bedroom is enough to reduce the problem to an acceptable level. An allergic child's room should be like a monk's cell—only a bed, and no dust-catching curtains, unwashed rugs, or other furnishings. Seal off the hot-air flue and use electric or steam heat. Clean only with a wet mop or oiled rag. Keep the door to the room shut, and the springs and mattresses enclosed in plastic coverings. Pillows should be foam rubber and blankets nonallergenic. No birds, cats, or dogs should be allowed in the house. (Turtles or fish are okay.) Avoid insect sprays or odoriferous substances. Toys should be washable or made of foam rubber.

If the child's symptoms are seasonal, suspect trees, grass, or weeds. If they are nocturnal, suspect the bed or bedroom. Some causes are simple to figure out, because the child is like a Geiger counter—aim his nose at the offending substances and see if he sneezes. Many allergic people have such complicated problems that the detective work of the allergist is necessary. Allergy testing is developing into a fairly accurate science, especially in determining sensitivity to pollens, molds, and animal danders. Testing for food sensitivities is helpful, but the elimination diet is the most reliable method.

The allergist takes a history, does testing, tries elimination. If no improvement is noted he will begin a vaccine injection program. If he is wise, he says, "Give me three years and maybe he'll be better."

It is amazing to me—and to most mothers—how a child's irritable disposition and sluggish behavior disappear soon after embarking on the proper allergy control regime. As I have pointed out, allergies are not only debilitating in themselves but may also lead to serious secondary complications such as bronchitis, ear infections (and deafness), skin infections (staphylococcus boils and skin scarring), nasal polyps, anal fissures, ulcers, and so on. Even worse, a mother may inadvertently lead her child into psychological problems because of her concern for his health. It is all too easy to turn him into a weakling, sissy, or hypochondriac, because every time he sniffles she asks, "Are you going to wheeze today?" If he coughs, she asks, "Did you get some phlegm out?" The child gets to be a navel (or nasal)—gazer and cannot be normal—his self-concern has been forced on him.

I have to emphasize the point that any child whose energies are consumed in coping with allergies can only feel less than perfect, and his behavior can disrupt the household. A chronic allergy victim usually looks malnourished with circles under his eyes, is somewhat pale, often open-mouthed, and droopy-looking. Controllable physical problems can lead to uncontrollable psychological ones. The mother is aware of his appearance and of course is constantly reminded by in-laws and neighbors that she ought to do something about his poor physical condition. This rankles most mothers who are already doing their best to rear their children properly, and they become nervous and distraught. It is normal to become resentful of the child's condition and appearance, when so much time and money have been devoted to improving his health. If you suspect your child may be putting you in this position, begin with food elimination tests and the "dust-free-room" battle plan outlined at the end of this chapter. Also refer to the Allergy Check List.

Control the allergy and you may control the child's irritable behavior. Control the allergy and you may be able to cut down serious secondary infections that could possibly lead to neurological damage. If your child is allergic to uncontrollable factors such as pollen in the air, you should take him to a specialist before fall and spring (the great sneeze times) come around again.

ALLERGY CHECK LIST

FOODS MOST LIKELY TO CAUSE TROUBLE

milk	pork
cottage cheese	green vegetables
ice cream	citrus fruits and tomatoes
chocolate	vitamins
wheat	spices
corn	garlic
fish	onions
eggs	nuts

SAFEST FOODS

veal	applesauce
beef	bananas
lamb	pears
rice	yellow vegetables
barley	

MOST COMMON INHALANTS CAUSING NASAL OR LUNG TROUBLE

housedust—usually a
mixture of molds,
fur, cottonseed

animal hair or dander
from cats and dogs,
birds, horses, pigs (in
upholstery)

cottonseed in furniture
and mattresses

pollens from trees in
spring, grass in spring
and summer, ragweed
in summer and fall

chemical irritants such as
sprays, deodorants,
cleansers

MOST COMMON CONTACTANTS ARE

rubber in pants and
elastic

plastic in toys, toilet
seats, bibs

wool in coats and
sweaters

synthetic fibers in
clothing

metal in rings and toys

makeup and deodorants

poison oak, ivy, and
sumac

Water, wood (untreated), and white cotton are usually safe.

INSTRUCTIONS FOR THE PREPARATION AND MAINTENANCE OF A DUST-FREE ROOM

All surroundings should be as free as possible from dusts of all kinds. Most people cannot control the dust conditions under which they work or spend their daytime hours, but everyone can to a large extent eliminate dust from the bedroom. These simple instructions will help you prepare and maintain a dust-free sleeping room:

CLEAN THE ROOM THOROUGHLY

1. Remove all furniture, rugs, curtains, and draperies from the room. Empty all closets.
2. Clean the walls, ceiling, and floors. Scrub the woodwork and floors in the bedroom and closets. Wax the floors.

KEEP IT FREE FROM DUST

1. Any flues that open into the room should be sealed. If you have hot-air heating, seal the opening with oil cloth and adhesive tape and use an electric heater. If this is not practical, then place a cotton screen over the hot-air outlet behind the grating, and change the screen frequently.

2. The furniture that has been removed from the room should be thoroughly cleaned before it is returned. The room should contain a minimum amount of furniture and furnishings. A wood or metal chair may be used (not upholstered). Use plain rag rugs and plain light curtains (both of which must be washed least once a week).

3. The room must be cleaned daily, and given a thorough and complete cleaning once a week. Clean the floor, furniture, tops of doors, window frames, sills, etc., with a damp cloth or oil mop. Air the room thoroughly. Then close the doors and windows until the child is ready to occupy the room.

4. Keep the doors and windows of this room closed as much as possible, especially when you are not using the room. Use this room for sleeping only. Dress and undress in another room.

BEDDING IS IMPORTANT

1. Scrub the bed (or beds). Scrub the springs.

2. Box springs, mattress, and pillows must be encased in dustproof coverings. These are impervious to dust, and keep the child from coming in contact with the harmful allergens that are present in all bedding material.

3. Be sure to clean the bed and encase the pillows, box springs, and mattress *outside of the bedroom* before they are returned to the room.

4. Do not use any kind of mattress pad. Sheets and blankets should be laundered weekly.

5. If there are two beds in the room, both of them must be treated as described above.

GENERAL SUGGESTIONS

1. Care must be taken to keep down the dust throughout the entire house. Go over all floors and furniture with a vacuum cleaner at frequent intervals—once daily if possible.

Following this, the house should be aired thoroughly. Cleaning must be done while the child is away from the house. Use a damp or oiled cloth to avoid raising the dust.

2. Pets, birds, and animals must be kept out of the house. Cats and dogs should be particularly discouraged.

3. Avoid cosmetics, perfumes, insect sprays, or powders, and odoriferous substances such as camphor, tar, etc.

4. The child should not go into any room while it is being cleaned. He should be careful not to handle objects that are covered with dust, such as books, boxes, or clothing that have been stored in shelves or cupboards over a long period of time. He should be kept away from attics and closets.

5. Keep out of the room all toys that will accumulate dust. Use only unstuffed, washable toys.

6. Keep bedroom door closed. Place flap at bottom.

8 ◆◆◆◆◆◆

STEPPING OUT OF
THE NEST

"It seems like yesterday he was a helpless little baby."

By the time a child has reached the age of six, his parents have usually seen him through the childhood diseases and have come to accept him and love him in spite of his faults (which were inherited from the wrong side of the family, of course). His personality is pretty well established. The job to be faced during the next period of his life is to get him educated, exposed to a certain amount of cultural advantages and see that he develops physically through participation in some athletic activity. The boy becomes a man and the girl a woman.

Some things in a child's life are uncontrollable, but it is possible to manipulate the environment to a considerable extent. Everything the mother does for her child is aimed toward the goal of pushing him out of the nest some day. She practices some amateur genetics by marrying a man who has the qualities she would like to see in her children. She tries to live in a neighborhood where she will be comfortable. She may be limited by financial considerations, but she wants to be near a good school. A few PTA meetings or neighborhood coffees will tell her if she is properly placed. Many women *have* to relate to the other mothers on the block; if they cannot or find them forbidding because of the different social or intellectual level, they may have to move. Working mothers, or families who work and play well together, may find neighborhood attitudes and pressures of minor importance and can be comfortable anyplace.

If a mother has some choice, and her husband does not insist on a certain "address" for business or status purposes, she will settle in an area where she senses social and intellectual similarities. She can only be comfortable in this environment and knows instinctively that she can rear her child more effectively if she is free of anxieties. Roughly then, the general intellectual tone of a school is determined by the families who cluster in its district—as flocks of birds will group together. One young professional I know told me that he must have lived in the wrong neighborhood as a child. To be popular with his neighborhood friends he did what seemed appropriate—damaged property and failed to achieve in school. When his family moved to a different neighborhood, his new friends used their energy in school and sports; he shifted gears, grades went up, vandalism disappeared.

The classroom teacher is usually more efficient if the IQ range of her class is narrow (say 90-110.) If she has a wide scatter to teach (a couple of 130's in a class of mainly 100's), she may not have enough time or energy to keep the bright from boredom. Since all children should receive an optimum education special plans have to be made for the very dull or very bright at the extremes of the class IQ curve.

If you are comfortably adjusted in the "right" neighborhood, and your child collapses in tears each day after school, you first suspect the school is too hard on him. With the help of your doctor, you have to determine if your child's problem is a low IQ, hypermotor behavior, illness, neurosis, neurological defect —or simply a too-tough teacher. Try calling the mothers of other children in the class to see if more than 50 percent are having trouble. If only 10 to 20 percent of the class is, then he needs a check-up. Hopefully, he has a minor treatable physical problem like wax in his ears, anemia, defective vision, or chronically infected tonsils. On the other hand, if most of his class is symptomatic then his teacher needs to get some feedback from the mothers so she can lighten the class load. But if you don't go through the right channels—child, teacher, doctor—and instead give the principal or school administration a hard time, the school may take out its wrath on the child.

Many children have a built-in prodding device, whether inborn or foisted on them by parents with high-achievement goals. These children are often overly serious, driven. They are more prone to stomach ulcers or at least stomachaches. They try hard to please, but cannot live up to the standards they have set for themselves. Even though they are always disappointed in their own work, teachers love these children for being eager, and responsive, doing their homework, and bringing fresh ideas and extra projects to school. But they are unpopular with their classmates because they are teachers' pets and get top grades. This isolates them socially and, because they are sensitive to start with, they get depressed and tearful. They either let their work go for the sake of becoming popular, or develop symptoms of tension or outright behavior problems. At any rate, they may have to accept their status as misfits unless they are sent to a private school (where many such children are sent). This solution is of course impossible for the poor family.

Now consider a child with *average* intelligence and drives, born or adopted into an academically oriented, intellectually competitive family. This child can never achieve the level he suspects is important for love in this home. His parents may reassure him that "we love you for what you are," but he still knows he is not up to the household standards. Again, frustration-anxiety symptoms result. This child should be induced to seek nonacademic pursuits in which he may feel successful. Doing average or poor school work, he will at least be able to tolerate his parents' sighs if he's winning on other fronts. (This desire for well-roundedness may in part explain the vicious aggression parents demonstrate at Little League and school athletic programs. They realize their child needs to win a little, and they help in the only way they know: "Drive!" "Go!" "Kill 'em!")

Tragically, certain children are produced with less-than-adequate mental capacity. If a child's IQ is markedly lower than his parents', then it is obvious—you can see and accept it. But when his intelligence is down just enough to disturb academic achievement, parents are afraid or reluctant to accept it and may become defensive and overprotective. Usually a mother suspects the problem before the doctor does, but she cannot put her worry into words. The doctors knows she is right, but he cannot define the problem either, because the clues are not foolproof. He knows if he makes a flat-footed statement like, "He is retarded," the mother will call twenty years later to say that he has just graduated from Yale *cum laude*.

A child's ability may not be challenged until he is about five or six years old and cannot handle his schoolwork. Often concurrent behavior problems may mask his real intelligence, making him *seem* retarded or at least immature. Most school systems have—or should have—psychological testing services available to help teacher, parents, and administrators decide IQ levels, grade assignments, and possible psychological and neurological problems. Teachers can often pinpoint children's problems more quickly than mothers, even to the point of recognizing the difficulty as low IQ, as psychological, or as neurological.

The mother of a less-than-adequate child is loath to accept teachers' and psychologists' decisions because of the implication that she has done something wrong. She will shop around for other authorities, to confirm that her child is "normal but sensitive," "a late bloomer," or "introverted." Such judgments may all be true, but until better methods are found to evaluate mental adequacy, she should rely on the teachers and psychologists.

In a class of twenty-five to forty there will be at least one child who is retarded—at least relative to the others. There will be at least one who is hypermotor, one who has a neurological problem and/or dyslexia, and at least one who is psychologically crippled. These children often find each other and begin to needle and aggravate the teacher and disrupt the class. The teacher uses isolation, threats, punishment, rewards—occasionally successfully. Big schools usually find it most efficient to put these children in a special class with a patient, long-suffering teacher who can motivate each with individual attention and allow him success at his own level. Surrender is the implication when a mother sees her child put into such a class; she feels he is "branded." But the wise mother will soon see her happy child having a successful learning experience, now winning more than he is losing.

The distraught parents of a retarded child have to face a similar decision when they find they cannot cope with his antics at home—he is so wearying, physically and emotionally. Overtly or covertly, the average family rewards its children for academic skills. The retarded child may sense this and become frustrated in school *and* at home when he cannot achieve. In this case, he will do better if he is placed in a suitable institution. He will be happy because he can compete with *some* success, and chances are his behavior will improve.

In the case of a severely retarded child, no doctor should try to dictate a parent's best course of action. He should state the alternative routes and then let husband and wife make their own decision. The family who already has five normal children and then produces a mongoloid child may choose to institutionalize it at birth. But another mother may find great fulfillment in keeping her defective—and dependent—child at home. These solutions may not be right for a third mother with different needs; each has to make her own "comfortable" decision.

Let us assume that your comfortable children are comfortable in school. You must then decide about music, dancing, drama, and art lessons. Should your child join the Scouts, Campfire Girls, or YMCA programs? Remember that most children get enough mental and physical stimulation at school and need some free time to just stare into space, watch a bug crawl through the grass, or smell spring coming.

In any case, they drag their feet about beginning any new activity you initiate for them. Mostly, they fear failure. The wise instructor or den leader starts out with projects, tunes, dances, and sketches that give an immediate satisfaction of accomplishment. Success breeds success. As time goes on and skills develop, the goals can be postponed, but must be clearly outlined: the recital, the play, the exhibit, award night, and so on.

You should try to enroll your children in at least one extracurricular activity a year. There will come a time when your child's innate abilities and his appropriate activity coincide, and he will turn on by himself. Nothing will delight you more than being able to say you were instrumental in bringing out your child's talent. You must decide how much to push from the home front and you, your child, and his instructor have to come to some understanding of risks ahead. If the music teacher says he really has talent, you must carefully consider the pros and cons before opting in favor of hours of drudgery and practice. If he is happy more than he is miserable, the programs are geared at the right level.

The mother of a champion swimmer called me to ask if her son was being pushed too hard. "He swims fifty laps after school, comes home, eats dinner, vomits, swims fifty laps, comes home, vomits, studies, sleeps, swims fifty laps, comes home. eats breakfast, vomits, and goes to school."

It sounded to me like this was too much.

We are rarely asked what sport, physical activity, extracurricular activity or cultural pursuit parents should push. If a child is innately floppy and clumsy, his mother will sometimes enroll her in ballet, modern dance, or him in some sport requiring balance and agility. Depending on the instructor, the child might just do well and enjoy it. But usually this awkward kid hates it because he does poorly and does not want to be laughed at. Occasionally, physical examinations can detect some "soft" neurological sign indicating future trouble in sports. Awkwardness in climbing on the examining table, peculiar gait, knock knees, pronated ankles, or knees that bend backward all suggest neurological or orthopedic weakness that may or may not be overcome. At the doctor's suggestion, a wise mother should get off her child's back if a physical fitness program is too much for him. Most schools have a variety of programs, so by the time he is seven or eight he will know whether he is varsity material.

From five to sixteen years or so, a child's chief task is to work up to his academic potential. If he succeeds well, sports may be of secondary interest to him. If he is so-so about books but does well in sports, he may tolerate school as a necessary evil so he can get to the main job of winning athletically. If school *and* sports are a drag, postschool music or art may help him retrieve his self-respect. If the boy has a bad eye and no depth perception, and all the fellows are playing tennis or baseball, he will be miserable—he should be swimming. I worry about the child who is maladroit, does poorly in school, and does not even have a record player, drum set, or stamp collection.

Schools should gear their sports and physical education to the child and not to his age. I believe all should be taught the importance of fitness and should be made to learn to swim, but not every kid needs to be able to do five push-ups just because he is in the fourth grade. When academic utopia arrives, there will be separate programs for the thin, the fat, the medium and the slob.

Most authorities feel that contact sports such as football are not suitable for the growing child. The child with "relaxed" ligaments or poor muscle development obviously runs greater risk of injury to his growing bones. The boy with these problems is often a disappointment to an athletically oriented father. What you intuit about your child's ability should be documented by the doctor's examination—and then your child can be encouraged in the direction of his most probable success. We are all proud of our country's gold-medal athletes, but there is a lot of room for poets, artists, actors, musicians, model builders, cooks, and visionaries. There is a sports page in every paper, but it would not be worth reading if there were not good sedentary journalists to write the copy.

When the six- to twelve-year-old comes in for a checkup, one of the first questions we ask is, "How's he getting along in school?" If the answer is, "Fine," and the examination is negative, we do not probe around too much. If the child can adjust to the aggravations of school in a healthy way, he will probably do all right later on. His "relating to his peer group" may be more important than the factual education he gets. Of course, if we ask the *child* how he is doing, he will say "Okay," no matter *how* well he is getting along. But his smile or tone will give away his real feeling. Fortunately for parents (and for us also), 80 percent of children are doing well enough at school to have themselves a happy childhood. They are succeeding somewhere.

The budding adolescent can trip an unwary mother. Grades may drop, behavior becomes sullen and speech abusive. You may hope he has infectious mononucleosis, but he usually doesn't. At this age, the slightest personality quirks seem to become major neurotic traits. We can sometimes ease the family over these hurdles, depending on how comfortable we are with the teenage group. Many pediatricians become insecure when they see one curly pubic hair, and shoot the patient off to the internist, as if by maturing, he had broken a promise. Check the length of the doctor's examining tables; this would be a clue as to his top age level.

We usually say a child should have a checkup annually from

two on. Once he is six, however, his mother is often the best judge of when he should be examined. She knows if something is wrong. Pediatricians listen for key words and phrases. When they hear them, lights flash on with directional arrows pointing to agencies, psychologists, ophthalmologists, nose and throat specialists, and educators.

The chart at the end of this chapter may give some insight into how we doctors do our work.

Needless to say, only part of a child's education comes from the classroom or the Scout troop. At the same time, the child is picking up all kinds of clues from his parents as to what it means to be an adult. Eventually, boys tend to pair off with their fathers, and girls with their mothers. But the pediatrician rightly feels that Mother is all-important for both sexes in the first two years. The father planted the seed, supplied half the genetic background, and after the child is born is supposed to stick around to support him and his mother. The wise husband, secure in his role, allows his wife to set the tone. He should offer to help, but he is expected to be a little clumsy with diapers, bottles, and other maternal chores.

A woman usually knows—correctly—when to give in when a child is protesting about schoolwork or mealtimes. A father has preconceived ideas; he is unwilling to compromise with his previously announced stand. "He will eat all his supper." (It is forced down and soon returned.)

A mother knows her under–two-year-old better because she is more skilled in nonverbal communication. Once the child begins to make more sense, his father shows more interest.

Mothers rarely mention their husbands to me (for a variety of reasons) until their son is maturing. Then it is, "How can I get his father to show an interest? This boy needs him." However a man cannot easily try to be a "pal" after twelve years of silence. (In some families it is fortunate that the father is not home much; if his wife and children got to know him better, it would wreck his image. One psychologist suggested that if the workweek were shortened, the divorce rate would soar.) When father suddenly takes his son to dinner to tell him the facts of life (at Mom's insistence), the venture fails because two embarrassed strangers will always have trouble communicating. A son may respect his father more if he did not get too close and chummy. Therefore, don't force your husband into a role he cannot play. He cannot fake an interest in the child. Young people despise our deceit and hypocrisy more than anything else. If it is a boy, you, of course, hope his father will "teach" him to be a man—strong, somewhat aggressive, mature, athletic. But most boys have an innate drive to be men, and girls to be women. If a father is frequently absent from a family made up of girls and a mother, how does a boy baby know enough to be masculine? The father didn't teach him; the genetic structure told him.

In my office I once had a rocking chair with a detachable arm. When a two-year-old boy sat down and discovered that the arm pulled out of its socket, he almost invariably tried to replace it. A girl of the same age would hand it to her mother and say, "Fix." Boys from age five on will ask, almost beg, to use my stethoscope or my light. Boys notice sounds of motors first. Boys bite, throw, have more physically aggressive play. Girls are domestic, and more verbal in expressing frustration. Though some feel this is because the sexes are treated differently from birth, I think a child initiates the behavior according to either male or female genetic promptings. Then his playmates and parents reinforce him.

Many fathers feel guilty because they are not able to take their sons on hunting trips, teach them how to box or enjoy playing ball with them. They are simply not comfortable doing this, but have heard if they do not, their son will surely become a fairy. Some 5 percent of all males will become homosexual, but for a variety of reasons: genetic aberrations, overly dominant mother, punitive father, etc. But the father's inability to play the role of the male stereotype is *not* necessarily the cause.

The mother's demonstration of her love and respect for the father will do more to lead a son to manhood than the father's ability to kill a deer. The child will easily move out of his secure, comfortable nest because you have let him be successful somewhere else.

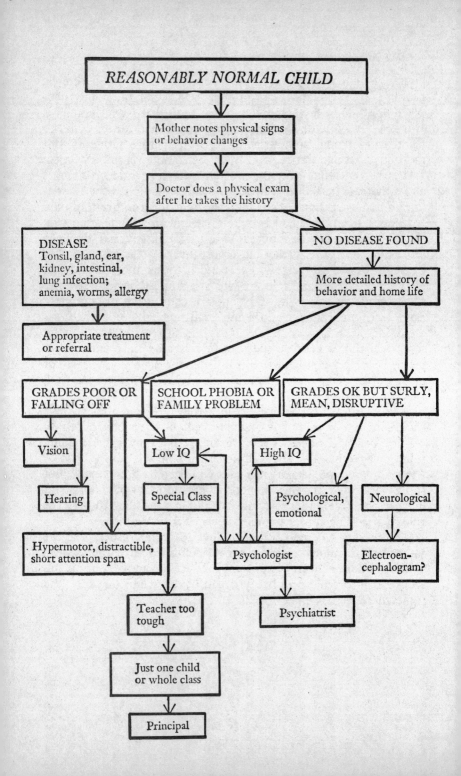

9 ◆◆◆◆◆

TELLING YOUR SUB-TEEN CHILD ABOUT SEX

"Well ... um ... er ... ah ...."

If your parents were happy and relaxed in dealing with your questions about sex, chances are you won't have too much trouble communicating with *your* child. Schools can teach reproductive anatomy, but telling it like it is about sex is still mainly your job. Mother is usually the one who comes in handy for the questions that occur out of the classroom.

When it comes to sex, your child wants straight, honest answers. If he says a loaded word and you blush, go to pieces, or hit him for being dirty-minded, he will either use the word again to bug you, or build a wall between you on the subject of sex. You must be ready. You must give answers that are *fast*, *honest*, and in a language *suitable* to his age.

A mother told me of her six-year-old daughter's loud query in the grocery store.

"What's that?"

"It's a box of sanitary napkins," the mother answered, trying to remain calm, although the store seemed to be awfully crowded.

"What are they for?"

"Well," said the mother, her knuckles white on the shopping cart handle, "grown up women use them."

Her daughter's next statement indicated that the lesson in mother-daughter communication was over for that day.

"Where's the cookies?"

The point is that the mother answered the question immediately and honestly and gave an answer that was just right for a six-year-old. This mother also indicated to her child that she was willing to answer her questions. This kind of parent-child dialogue must be kept alive.

A warm realtionship of mutual trust and respect, coupled with firm limits established in early childhood, will determine your child's ability to cope with his hormones later on. A child needs an adult to test out his feelings and to guide him safely through the times of turmoil. He needs a home base while he experiments with different life styles. (The school's role is that of an ice-breaker, and it should not be expected to take complete and unsupplemented responsibility. Subjects will be brought up at school that can and should be comfortably explored at home.)

Children do not have to know everything. Sometimes we tell them more than they want to know. Start simply and easily with facts and ideas that are not traumatic to *you*. You will find it easier if you proceed gradually.

Age two to three years. Your son is getting taller and his stomach is flatter. He discovers his penis. It itches. He scratches it or rubs it against the mattress in a suggestively sexual way. Your first thought is that he is "over-sexed" or worse—mentally deranged in some obscure, untreatable way. Your first impulse is to smack him, but you decide to play it cool. You ask objectively, "Does your penis itch?"

"Yes," he answers, without embarrassment (unless *you* show it.)

"Well," you say, "maybe you're drinking too much orange juice or that new bubble bath is irritating you."

You should look on his "fooling" with himself as clinically as possible, with no more emotion than you would show if the itchy spot were on his elbow.

You are seven months along in your second pregnancy and your three-year-old daughter says, "Why are you so fat?"

"Your brother or sister is growing inside me and in a few months will be big enough to live outside," is a good answer. "Besides," you might add indignantly, "I am *not* fat; I've merely lost my waistline."

"Can I have a baby, please?" she pleads.

"Not now, dear," you reply. "You'll have to wait until you're grown up and settled in a home where you can take care of a baby properly. But you can help me with this one and see how you like mothering. We can have fun together."

By this simple exchange, your child has learned a few facts about human beginnings and hopefully has gotten an idea about adult responsibility and our duty to the next generation. Your calm response indicates that sexual relationships and pregnancy are as normal as other bodily functions. You have suggested, that being an adult female is a pretty good goal for a girl. You have allowed her to talk and ask. She will come back again and seek you out.

Age four to six years. The neighborhood witch is on the phone saying that she has just caught your four-year-old son in her garage looking at her four-year-old daughter's "privates." She is incoherently screaming about "nasty boys," "rape," calling the police, needing a psychiatrist, and moving off the block. You know you cannot settle her hash in two minutes over the phone. (You also suspect that her girl is a flirt and a tease and will probably grow up to be a prostitute.) Instead, you promise to 1) talk to your son, 2) have your husband punish him, and 3) call the pediatrician. Do not be too angry with her for misinterpreting childhood curiosity, mad at your son for putting you into this embarrassing spot, or upset with yourself for not supervising him more carefully. He will arrive home with a mixed expression of fear and puzzlement.

"What happened?" your voice cracks.

"Oh, we were playing doctor," he tells truthfully.

"Was she sick?" you stall.

"No, just checking." He begins to leave.

"Let's talk. Were you checking to see if she was a boy or a girl? Is that why you looked?"

"Well, ah. . ."

"You have a penis. Right?"

"Yeah."

"Girls don't have one; they have an opening called a vagina. All right?" You might draw a picture. "It's the same the world over. Some mothers don't like their daughters looked at. Please respect their wishes. The doctor may do it because it is part of his job. If you want more information, just ask me, and we'll get a book with better pictures. Okay?"

"Okay."

Your six-year-old girl has never asked a question about parts of the body, differences between sexes or how life begins. She may know it all, but you cannot be sure. An opener might be:

"Ann, I'm curious to know if you know where babies come from."

Ann: "Out of the mother's tummy."

You: "How?"

Ann: "Through the belly button."

You: "That's not right. It comes out through her vagina, the front opening on her bottom. Who told you it was the belly button?"

Ann: "John, a smart kid in our class. He says he knows everything because his dad is a doctor."

You: "Well, that's why we go to school—to learn. And you can always ask me questions, too. I know some things John doesn't know. If I don't know, we can look them up together."

Unless she asks more, let the subject drop for the time being. But in six months or a year ask again by trying the next step.

You: "How did the baby get inside me?"

Ann: "You swallowed it."

You: "No, Daddy puts the seed in the vagina. The seed meets the egg which is already in there, and the baby starts to grow. Everyone in the whole world started that way."

You might have to wait six months for *that* to sink in but if there are no questions for another year, try again. If you are nervous or shy, it will be harder the longer you wait.

Your nine- to twelve-year-old son comes home and tries out a four-letter, Anglo-Saxon word that he learned from an eighth grader. Explain, when you catch your breath, that these are terms ignorant people use to embellish their meager conversation. Make sure he knows two or three "acceptable" words to substitute for every "bad" one. If he tries to shock you, tell him it is old stuff to you. But watch your own language. Be sure he does not hear you use one of *his* favorite words the next time you drop the soufflé on the kitchen floor.

Your response to your children's feelings and questions about sex might be compared to the comments you would make about their artwork. Instead of asking with a sneer, "What's that?" you turn the child on with, "Hey! Great! Tell me the story of the picture." If your child is six to nine years old you might ask, "What do you think of the way God lets us have babies? Do you think there is a better way?"

As your child gets older, his school may or may not provide adequate information. Most schools have a film on menstruation which is shown to sixth, seventh, and eighth-grade girls in Home Economics. The film is a good one, but if the girls do not see it on the very first day of their very first menstrual period, it doesn't have much impact. If they have already had a couple of periods, they're old hands and think, "I know all about that stuff." If they have not yet had a period they think, "Who cares?" Still a child learns some of these emotionally-charged facts better in a classroom. Make sure your school has embarked on such a program involving *each* grade level from kindergarten on. If it is not yet a part of the curriculum, get the P.T.A. to push it.

Keep up your running dialogue. Your child needs to feel reasonably comfortable with you in any discussion of sex. I know some parents who are a little unsure of themselves and fear they will be too embarrassed to answer their children's questions properly. I suggest they go to a book store which has a pretty complete selection for each age group. But remember: when you get a book that is just right for your six, seven, or twelve-year-old, you do not just hand it to him and say, "Read this. We're going to have a quiz next week." The child will feel you are trying to educate him, and naturally refuse. It often works better to hide it in the top of your closet. The child is then sure to find it and read it, thinking it is taboo.

DO's

Mothers and children bathing together encourage laughter, warmth, and a sense of belonging. Everyone gets cleaner and saves water. You might as well be in the tub with your children; you will get just as wet outside. This provides an opportunity for natural questions about anatomy to be asked. When your child gets to be five or so he may want to bathe alone. Respect his wishes. As a child grows older, he should be taught to knock before entering a bedroom or bathroom. You may not care if he sees you naked, but he should be trained to respect the privacy of others and want it for himself.

Your child's curiosity about body functions should be satisfied as much as possible at home or he will seek the answers elsewhere. He learns to feed himself because you feed yourself. He becomes toilet trained because you use the toilet. He respects others because you do. Encourage his interest with factual answers.

DONT's

Don't let your child play with another considerably older child. The older child who enjoys this relationship is usually deficient in the ability to find friends his own age and likes to impress younger kids with his "superior," if misguided, knowledge.

Don't be punitive with your son if he brings pictures of nude women to his room or shares them with classmates. Try to be "objective." (*i.e.* "Did you know that the left breast is usually larger than the right?") If you make sexy pictures completely taboo for him, he will think they are more important than they are. Accept them as a lusty interest, but suggest discretion and moderation.

Don't assume your son's sexual interests are something he has been taught by his father. This interest is characteristic of the male of the species and cannot be eliminated.

One important thing that your child should remember is that sex was not discovered yesterday; it is a fact of life; a part of "maleness" and "femaleness." The normal, natural curiosity of the young child should be dealt with in a normal, natural matter-of-fact way so that it will not be diverted into morbid preoc-cupation. The repressed child will assume that sex gratification is the sole attribute of maturity.

A mother must direct her child's sexual curiosity into socially acceptable outlets—science, hobbies, literature—and divert his energies to sports, games, and art forms.

Later on, during bull session or hen parties, your child will be equipped with the correct words and definitions. If he has the facts straight, he can clear up someone else's misconceptions and avoid them himself.

Your ability to be comfortable with your child while this running dialogue is carried on from age two to twelve will in a large part determine how comfortable he is in dealing with his *own* sexuality when his glands start to function. He should develop language skills so he can put a few of his feelings into thoughts and deal with them more effectively. You must allow him to practice some of his naïve thoughts out loud without showing shock, scorn, or ridicule. He will respect you for not devaluating him. If you believe he's a sneak, he will assume that role; we usually encourage the behavior we expect from people.

The budding adolescent, somewhat overwhelmed by his new physical dimensions and his compelling chemistries, "asks" for limits and rules just as surely as does the two-year-old who runs into the dangerous street. Until he is able to place sex in its proper perspective in *his* own life style, he needs your trust and a few guidelines. Life has plenty of mysteries and topics for good, hard thought. Sex is one of them—an important part of life, but only a part.

10 ◆◆◆◆◆◆

THE MOTHER AS
DETECTIVE

*"I knew something was wrong; I could
feel it."*

Many a baby doctor's day is filled with caring for healthy
babies. After struggling to look beyond the wax at the normal
ear drum of a one-year-old, getting his last clean shirt saturated
with urine, he is unconvinced he is doing anything of great
moment. He gives shots and polio drops that a public health
clinic could dispense more cheaply. He comforts mothers who
talk incessantly over the phone about trivial problems. "He had
a loose stool." "He sneezed." "May I use applesauce?" He often
seems to be the clearing house for syndromes but never the
ultimate authority: for a rash, see the dermatologist; for a hernia,
see the surgeon; for an eye problem, see the ophthalmologist.
Some parents really know how to hurt us when they call and
say, "My child has an ear infection; can you recommend a good
nose and throat specialist?" This would indicate that the pediatrician's training and his practice expectations are different from
what he finds when he opens his private office. Either his training had the wrong emphasis, or his personality is not suited to
the many nit-picking aggravations, or his patients do not have
the diseases he would like to treat.

I am writing this at ten o'clock on a Saturday night. A woman has just called because her three-month-old is rejecting solid foods. She needs to know if solids are so important that she must continue to force them into her combative baby. I know she felt it was an emergency or she would not have called. I couldn't get upset about her poor timing because I recognized that she was so insecure that she needed immediate reassurance. She was waving a red flag, just to tell me to pay attention and throw a little confidence her way.

Your pediatrician should guide you in acquiring the necessary confidence to rear your child. This is ultimately your responsibility, not his—he wants you to accept it, but he can help by giving you the benefit of his knowledge and objectivity. For today's mothers there is a whole new set of universal truisms or "new wives' tales." You need to be armed with knowledge and new perspectives in health and medicine. You need a value system which permits you to put daily events in proper perspective.

In this chapter are some medical dilemmas you may not know how to handle. Some of these problems are so insignificant you may be embarrassed to ask your doctor. Some of them you should know about simply because they are important and require his advice. Still others are very serious, and you should turn the whole problem over to him. Frequently you and your pediatrician will be able to work together as a team. If armed with enough facts, you will be a more confident mother and will need to bother him less with nuisance calls. He in turn will feel less harrassed and can devote more time to you and your philosophy of child-rearing.

Against a background of mutual trust, periodic visits to your doctor give you both a chance to evaluate your philosophy. The doctor needs to find out what sort of a person you are— average, bright, nit-picker, calm, tense, or scared. The wise pediatrician wants you to rear your own child, but he needs to study you on a continuing basis so he can guide and direct (but not dictate) your child-rearing policies. I am convinced that any doctor who is dissatisfied with his profession must be unaware of the valuable role he plays in shaping a healthy family unit. What are the family's goals? How does the wife react to stress, disease, death? Why did one marriage fall apart under a pressure that united a different family? Our medical schools have only recently, because of student pressure, put emphasis on detecting a family's pulse rate. The intuitive doctor knows that any one problem needs different handling in different families.

Some doctors I know call a mother each day during a period of crisis as a morale booster. She needs friendly, sympathetic support which she may not be receiving from their husband or mother-in-law. Your doctor should at least have time to discuss family attitudes, how much time off you need, your husband's role, child spacing, educational needs, in-law interference, careers outside the home, and so on. It might turn out that *he* will be asking more questions than you do. He will be your private child-rearing computer, and you will know how to push the proper button to get what is right for you.

A stomachache in Mrs. M's house is very serious, but is only gas in one of Mrs. V's children. Mrs. E gets a plastic surgeon for a cut chin; Mrs. H puts tape on it herself. Both methods are right! You do *not* have to follow every suggestion a doctor makes, but only take home what is appropriate for your situation. Sometimes I say, "Do this," to an indecisive mother, and it works. Occasionally I will suggest all the alternatives and let the mother decide which is most appropriate.

As you and your doctor work together, you will learn to communicate well enough so that when real crises come you will know how to talk. A mother's description of how, what, and when is essential in solving her child's problem. The child is a part of her, an extension of herself. When changes occur, she feels, intuits, "smells" something wrong. Her problem is to relate her information in words. The doctor has to translate her message into terms that will spell out the right symptom in *his* frame of reference. For example:

Mother's Comment	*Doctor's Note Pad*
"He didn't finish his peas."	Anemia, sickness, too many peas
"His naps are fifteen minutes longer."	Up late, house less tense or noisy, outgrowing allergy
"When he did this before, he had an earache."	Mumps, flu, ear infection

This takes skill, training, and time. In my first year of practice, I felt any baby who cried more than twenty minutes a day had a milk allergy. I cringe to think of all the babies I put on soy bean milk. Now through a combination of questions, intuitions, and responses, I am more quickly able to decide that one might do better with a sedative; another with larger, more frequent feedings; another with having the bottle propped. A mother with several children is usually a "pro" at figuring out what the problem is—she has seen them all. But let us say you are starting out with your first child. Until you get acquainted with him, you will have difficulty recognizing just what is normal for him. The following section might answer a few of the questions you would be likely to call your doctor about. There are as many how-to-do-it's as there are what-to-do-about-it's. A larger selection of topics is classified in this book's "Quick Reference Directory" under *Emergencies, Diseases,* and *Conditions* so that you will be able to assign them the proper "worry" value.

CATEGORY I—"Be Reassured"

A. *Just home with the new baby*

Bathing is best done in a plastic dishpan. Use as little soap as possible.

Blood on the outside of a bowel movement is usually associated with a crack or fissure at the anal opening. Poking a dollop of petroleum jelly into the anal opening after each stool should control this in a few days.

A blue tinge to the lips and nails is due to extra red blood cells that have been inadequately oxygenated during quiet sleep following a full meal; the blueness should disappear when the baby starts crying.

A baby who *cries himself to sleep* is normal. Twenty minutes is about all of this anyone can stand, but some babies need to do this.

Cold hands and feet are related to circulation and not disease. Much of a baby's circulation is diverted to his intestinal tract to aid digestion. If the temperature of the room is 65-70° F., and his skin is warm in the middle of the back, he is all right.

Drinking water is not necessary, since milk is about 90 percent water. Most babies choke on it anyway. If he urinates three to five times a day, he is getting enough fluid.

Navel care can cause needless concern. Some dried up cord remnant usually adheres to the navel. If it gets too dry, the healing skin underneath will crack and bleed. Bathe it with soap (best with hexachlorophene) and water. Alcohol is okay, but it tends to dry it more. It is best to use an antibiotic ointment around the stump of the cord to keep it free of bacteria and soft and pliable. (Do the same with a circumcision wound.)

If he *sleeps all day and cries or fusses all night,* he has sleep reversal. Try to feed him every two to three hours in the day so he may get his 24-hour quota during the daylight hours. If he is breast-fed, he may be reacting to some food his mother is eating for supper (fish, garlic, cabbage, etc.). He may need to scream it out, or may need a sedative.

A *swelling on side of the head* (cephalohematoma) is a collection of blood and serum on the outside of the skull bone, not a depressed fracture.

A *swollen scrotum* is usually due to a hydrocele, a harmless collection of fluid. It should stay the same size; if not, it may be a hernia.

Thumb-sucking after a full meal can be solved with a pacifier. Some babies like to suck. Let them.

Tongue-tie is a short, tough membrane between the floor of the mouth and the underside of the tip of the tongue. The only problem the child will have is in licking stamps; only rarely does one need clipping.

B. *He is three weeks old or so*

Belly bands (to hold the navel in) are a waste of time and do no good.

Cereal is often rejected at this age. Forget it and try again next month. Rice or barley is safest.

Constipation is the formation of hard, dry stools that are difficult to pass. Infrequent stool passage is not constipation; breast-fed babies may have only one or two bowel movements a week, but these are usually soft. Real constipation may be helped by changing the milk. Extra water does little good; he will only urinate more. Dark Karo in the milk (one to three teaspoons per bottle), prune juice, or milk of magnesia (one-half to one teaspoon in one or two bottles a day) may relieve it.

Cradle cap is related to pimples (see below) and usually responds to mineral oil and gentle brushing after shampooing.

If *DPT shots* were started and then two months went by, you don't have to start again. Just go ahead, but *get* them.

On the *first outing* at any time of the year, avoid sudden temperature and humidity changes. When going from house to car in winter, put a receiving blanket loosely over his face so he may rebreathe his own warm air.

Small pimples that develop over the forehead, chin, scalp, nose, and shoulder blades are a condition of plugged oil glands called *seborrhea*—just like adolescent acne. They will last a month, look terrible, and then scale off. Mineral oil is appropriate, not baby oil—some babies are sensitive to the perfume in the latter.

Vitamins are necessary. Many milks have vitamins added. There is no harm done if you wait until the one-month checkup and ask your doctor for free samples to see which tastes better. Some forgetful parents give seven times the usual daily dose once a week. Fluoride is usually begun with vitamins.

Watery, runny nose may be the result of a cold or hay fever. If it lasts a week, it is a cold. If it lasts longer and he is still sneezing, it is an allergy. Remove cats and dogs from the house; feather pillows, down comforters, and wool blankets from his bed, and read Chapter 8.

CATEGORY II—These problems need a doctor's attention within a few days.

Anemia usually develops slowly in an older baby who is drinking only milk. He usually is pale and tired and refuses solids—the very foods that would correct this iron-poor diet.

Constipation, if unrelieved by diet change, may need to be checked by an X ray or thyroid test.

Eczema usually occurs on the cheeks, the elbow creases, and behind the knees. Diet change and special ointments are necessary to control this weepy, scaly, red, itchy rash.

Hearing loss can usually be detected at home by testing the three-month-old's responses with bells or whistles.

Purulent matter in eyes may dry and occasionally cause them to become stuck shut. This is usually caused by conjunctivitis and is often related to a plugged tear duct. Like stagnant water, the tears cannot drain into the nose via this occluded canal, so infection sets in. Probably an eye antibiotic is needed.

A *red rash over the pubic and genital area*, often associated with white curdlike spots in the mouth, is usually thrush. Special medicine is required.

Scrotum swelling that comes out with crying and disappears with rest is a hernia. A truss is no good; surgery is needed.

Sleeping on the stomach in a knee-chest position, with toes pointing in, is comfortable because the baby took this position in the uterus. However, it puts pressure on the feet. If not corrected by manipulation, corrective shoes, or a brace, he will become pigeon-toed.

Stridor is noisy, throaty breathing on inspiration and expiration. In a content baby, it usually implies floppy vocal cords that will correct themselves.

Vomiting a number of feedings suggests that your child's stomach rejects milk or the fat in it. If he has bowel movements and urine, something is going through and you have time to experiment.

CATEGORY III—These are serious problems suggesting onset of grave diseases. Call your doctor immediately if you notice any of the following symptoms.

Asthma or tight wheeze on exhaling, especially if blue or cyanotic, needs immediate relief.

Bloody, jam-colored, or tarry stools mean internal hemorrhage.

Bloody urine may be caused by twenty or thirty conditions.

Blue discoloration or cyanosis may mean heart disease or pneumonia.

Continuous vomiting of all feedings, associated with scanty urine and infrequent, hard stools, probably means pyloric stenosis, an intestinal obstruction, or pressure on the brain.

Convulsions, with or without fever is a neurological problem,

Croup with fever that interferes with sleep and does not respond to steam and aspirin may require hospitalization.

Crying can mean pain. If the baby has a purulent discharge from his nose and refuses to suck on the bottle or cries when he does, this almost always means he has an ear infection. The vacuum created by the suction pulls on the inflamed eardrum, and he cries. If, however, he takes the bottle well but refuses to eat solids, this would indicate a sore throat, tonsillitis, canker sores, or teething.

Falls may not be serious, but the doctor should be notified.

Fever that does not respond to aspirin suggests a serious bacterial infection.

Lethargy with a loss of the sucking reflex may mean infection—meningitis, pneumonia, etc.

Pustules, boils, or abcesses in a baby are serious.

Swallowed poison, drugs, or foreign objects may or may not be dangerous; call the doctor.

Watery, *green stools* that are foul-smelling and accompanied by fever usually mean dysentery.

The alert mother who is attuned to her baby's general behavior patterns can detect deviations. She may even be able to figure out the problem. But if she wants to get the most from her doctor, she should allow him to do the diagnosis himself. The enjoyment of working with people, learning their strengths, weaknesses, and motivations, and helping them solve their problems are great personal satisfactions for doctors. But the most fascinating facet of medicine is the detective work required in diagnosing disease. We love the fun of piecing evidence together until a familiar pattern emerges which duplicates a pattern we stored away in medical school. We got a feeling for various bodily functions so that now, when we're faced with a sick patient, we almost automatically know what the problem is and how to solve it. The trick is to be a good diagnostician. Since 75 percent of disease states are diagnosed by history alone, since pediatrics is largely a talking profession, and since most children have but one disease at a time, it would follow logically that pediatrics should be a very fulfilling profession, if making the diagnosis is the doctor's chief reward. He needs to solve it, so let him.

If the mother calls to say her child has the measles, the doctor may agree that the child does. But because he was robbed of the opportunity to play his part, he may also try to disprove the poor mother who was only trying to help. In fact, he may even find that the fever is due to the flu, the cough is due to post-nasal drip, and the rash is due to an allergy. (It can happen.)

The wise mother will call and simply say her child has a fever, a cough, and a rash. *Then* the doctor can say, "It's probably the measles." If she knows her child was exposed to measles two weeks previously, she will readily accept the diagnosis, and both she and the doctor will be satisfied.

The patient who provides the accurate history usually gets the accurate diagnosis. You have to assume that if your doctor graduated from medical school, and if you are afflicted with something that is written up somewhere in the medical text-books, then your statement of the onset of the present illness, its chief complaint, and your past history will fit a "gestalt" that the doctor has in his brain.

All through school and clinical training a doctor wrote up his case histories in a standard way. Because he is familiar with this mental format, you might try using it with him to see if you get quicker, more accurate results. For example:

A. *Chief complaint*: "My three-year-old boy says his right ear hurts."

B. *Present Illness*: "Two weeks ago he got a cold with a fever and a croupy cough. After three days, his fever went away and the cough got more phlegmy. I've been giving him aspirin (one grain for each ten pounds of body weight) every four hours, a decongestant, and steam at night. He seemed to be almost over it two days ago, and then his fever went up to 101° and the cough got tighter. The material from his nose turned thick and yellow. Now he says that his right ear hurts."

C. *Past history*: "He has had all his shots and has had about ten colds in his life. Three of them developed into ear infections."

D. *Family history*: "Both my husband and I had ear

trouble when we were young, until our tonsils were taken out."

The doctor is familiar with this kind of *coherent* description and responds to it much better than he does to miscellaneous information reported in a garbled fashion. A few more pointers:

(1) Don't be reluctant to talk to the nurse about the problem first. She may help, if it is something she can handle, and will get you to the doctor faster when it *is* an emergency. At least she will allow you to practice telling the story of the sickness—as a dry run—so you will be better able to communicate with the doctor.

(2) Call at an appropriate time. If the child is very sick, or if it is an emergency such as the four B's (blueness, breaks, burns, or bleeding), call immediately. If the sick, feverish child can get up and walk around, you usually can wait until office hours.

(3) Be courteous and honest. "I'm sorry to bother you after hours, but this just happened." "I just got home from work and discovered something was wrong." "I knew it could wait until morning, but my husband insisted that I call." "We are leaving tomorrow for Mexico and we have to find out before we go."

(4) Have a pencil and paper handy; also, have the druggist's phone number. *Write down* any instructions, and make sure you understand them. It would be smart to repeat them as they are given. It will save another phone call later to ask, "What did you say?" This is especially helpful since we doctors often assume that patients have a few basic medical concepts in mind. A few times, after ordering an "internal liquid antibiotic" for an ear infection, I later have discovered that the mother had put it in her child's ear instead of giving it by mouth.

If you play this game by the above rules, you should be deriving the maximum benefits from the doctor-patient relationship. This is supposed to make you more competent, more confident, and hence, a better mother. (I assume better mothers rear better children.) If you can keep from being hung up on a lot of picayune nonsense, you will build as much love and security into your home as is necessary to rear a mature, responsible adult. (You will know you are successful when your child becomes a pediatrician and writes a book.)

Think of your child as a guest in your house—sometimes unwelcome, often ungrateful, frequently messy, but always a challenge in the good sense of the word. Show him a way of life a little more fulfilling than the one your parents provided for *you*. Teach him the rules of society so he will operate comfortably within its limits, not hurt others, nor have too much anxiety himself. Let him live his own life—not yours through him. Allow him to be reasonably critical and a little defiant about the way our generation has done things. It takes many years to develop one of these cautious rebels.

BIBLIOGRAPHY

Abrams, A.L., *Imipramine in Enuresis;* American Journal of Psychology. 120:177 (1963).

Illingworths, R.S., *How to Help a Child Achieve His Best;* Journal of Pediatrics. 73:61-68 (July 1968).

Kosman, M.E., et al., *Chronic Drug Administration;* Clin. Pharmacology. 9:240-254 (Mar. Apr. 1968).

Millichap, J.G., *Drugs in Management of Hyperkinetic and Perceptually Handicapped Children;* Journal of A.M.A. 206:1527-1530. (Nov. 1968).

Poussaint, A.F., et al., *A Controlled Study of Imipramine;* Journal of Pediatrics. 67:283 (1965).

Schwartz M., et al. *Positive Spiking in EEG;* Journal of Pediatrics, 72: 678-682 (May 1968).

Silver, H., et al., *Milk Intolerance in Infancy;* Arch Dis. Child., 43:17-22 (Feb. 1968).

QUICK
REFERENCE
DIRECTORY

━◆━◆━◆◆━◆◆━

Section I

EMERGENCIES

Accidents in the home can frequently be prevented. The wise mother might get down on her hands and knees at the level of her accident-prone, one- to three-year-old child and scoot around on the floor. See what attractive, low-down nuisances there are in the house, such as detergents under the sink, bottles of kerosene and gasoline, various sharp objects. Make sure your baby cannot climb onto high furniture or cabinets. Remove doors from unused refrigerators, and have suitable locks or combinations on the medicine closet (see also *Wounds* and *Head Injuries*.) Electric wall sockets should be covered. Always, *always* disconnect appliances from the wall socket; terrible mouth burns result when a toddler puts the "hot" end of an appliance cord in his mouth. Everyone should strap his child into the seat of a car when traveling; in an automobile collision, a child's light body frequently ricochets through the interior of the car like a Ping-Pong ball.

Appendicitis is an inflammation of the appendix, which in most people is found in the lower right area of the abdomen. If the inflammation is great enough, the appendix abcesses and ruptures, causing peritonitis. The trick is to diagnose appendicitis while the appendix is still intact, and get the surgeon to remove the dirty thing. It is now well-documented that appendicitis attacks can run in families; if parents had appendicitis when they were children, their children are more likely to develop it. I have seen it occur in twins within a few months of each other. Good rules to remember are: (1) appendicitis feels like the worst gas pain you have ever had, but it does not go away. (2) If you have a good bowel movement and the pain does *not* go away, it is probably appendicitis.

BEE STINGS cause more deaths than snake bites. People can be severely allergic to bee venom, and for some reason, adolescent males react more severely than anyone else. You should have antihistamines available to give immediately after the bite of any stinging insect. This sometimes reduces the swelling, itching, and pain that develop anywhere from a few hours to a whole day later. But the person who has violent reaction such as generalized hives, swelling in the throat, or fainting, usually requires adrenalin, and/or oxygen from a doctor. If a person has had such a generalized reaction he should get immunizing shots to protect himself.

BLUE DISCOLORATION or cyanosis means that not enough oxygen is getting into the system. It implies that there is some obstruction that prevents oxygen from reaching the blood stream. There may be an obstruction in a small baby's nose and he will be unable or unwilling to breathe through his mouth. He may have an infection in or a congenital anomaly of his throat or windpipe that prevents the easy inflow of air into his lungs. He may have a collapsed lung, pneumonia, or some problem that reduces the area of functioning lung tissue; or a heart anomaly where the unoxygenated blood is mixed with fresh, or where not enough blood is going through the lungs to become properly oxygenated. The nervous system suffers the most from lack of oxygen, and if prolonged or severe, this can result in brain damage. The obvious answer is to relieve the condition that is producing the lack of oxygenated blood and/or to give the patient increased amounts of oxygen. If the condition appears suddenly, it is a real emergency. The most important thing to do, besides calling the doctor, is to get someplace—such as a hospital emergency room or a doctor's office—where there is oxygen equipment. The local fire station usually has this and this is often the easiest place to get to and find relief.

BROKEN BONES are often quite obvious when they occur in an

arm or leg. They need professional care. The patient should be transported with suitable splinting to a hospital or doctor's office.

The easiest bone to break, however (and also one of the most rapid ones to heal), is the clavicle or collarbone. This injury usually results from a fall in which the patient strikes his shoulder. The collarbone—which lies between the shoulder and the upper part of the chest—cracks or splinters, and the bone ends override. Usually there is a tender lump at the site of the break. The next most common fracture is the broken ankle, which is sometimes confused with a sprain. (Some sprains are actually more serious than breaks because of the torn ligaments.) Fractures of the anklebone sometimes heal with very little splinting.

A fall on the outstretched hand may result in a fracture of the wristbone and give a characteristic "silver fork" deformity. This may not be too obvious, but in a child it may involve the growth center of the bone. If a fracture is suspected, careful X rays should be taken because of the need for proper positioning of the bones while healing. Perhaps the most effective "splinting" method that can be done at home is to use a rolled-up newspaper, blanket, or even a pillow to softly support the break. The point of careful splinting is to prevent a simple fracture from becoming compound—that is, having the bone end push through the skin. This latter condition may result in infection, which complicates healing.

A subluxation or partial dislocation of the radius bone at the elbow is not uncommon between the ages of one and three. This usually is sustained by the two-year-old who wants to go one way; his mother gives a tug on his outstretched arm. The bone is pulled out of position and immediately the child screams and lets his arm hang uselessly at his side. Any attempt to flex the elbow or move the forearm results in extreme pain. There is a maneuver that brings this back in position, but it must be done under medical supervision. X rays usually do not reveal this condition, but the position of the arm and the history of onset are diagnostic.

BURNS should be treated immediately, even before the doctor is summoned, by immersing the affected part in ice water—not just cold water, but ice water. If it is a hand or a foot, some ice in a bucket of water will do. If the extremity is kept in from one to four hours, the cold may keep a first-degree burn from becoming a second, or a second from becoming a third. If the burned area is on the body, an icepack can be made from a wet washcloth with ice in it, perhaps covered with some sort of plastic, and a big towel on top to hold it in place. Again, leave it on from one to four hours. Make sure the frigid water reaches the skin. This usually soothes the pain and somehow interferes with the formation of poison or toxin produced by burned tissue.

CONVULSIONS of a generalized nature occur in about 5 percent of those children who are hit suddenly with a high fever. Convulsions are frightening, but usually respond to temperature control and sedation. They seem to be an inherited tendency, are common between one and three years of age, and almost never lead to epilepsy in later life.

CROUP is a common childhood affliction. It usually appears rather dramatically in the middle of a winter night, when the air outside is clear and cold. The air in the house is usually dry, and this may trigger the attack.

Usually the child awakens suddenly between midnight and one o'clock, clawing the air, choking, and barking. The mother at first thinks the dog's been frightened until she realizes that the racket is coming from the nursery. She is usually quite frantic because her child seems scared to death, but after twenty minutes of being upright and inhaling steam, he should be relaxed and quiet. Because most drugstores are closed at that time of night, the best cough syrup is a mixture of equal parts of gin, lemon juice, and honey. For the twenty- to forty-pound child, a teaspoonful is usually adequate to cut and loosen the phlegm and to reduce anxiety for all concerned.

Croup is considered to be basically a virus affliction, although allergies and bacteria may play their parts. It almost invariably lasts for three nights, and if under the influence of steam, the victim can sleep for an hour or two in between the strangling, then he is all right. However, if his croup lasts longer than three days, or if twenty minutes of steam inhalation does not relax him enough to allow him to sleep, then he needs professional attention. One severe type of croup, almost always accompanied by a temperature of 103° or more, is due to bacterial infection. In this case, thick, tenacious, purulent matter occludes and swells up the vocal cords to the point where the child has to fight desperately for air. He may need hospitalization, oxygen, and perhaps even a tube inserted surgically into the windpipe (a tracheotomy). If his air is severely restricted, the child will become blue or cyanotic, and of course this may do some damage to his nervous system.

Some children develop a croupy sound after they have had a cold for a few days and have developed a secondary bacterial infection. Thick, tenacious material drips down into the windpipe, usually at night. If this is a chronic, recurring condition, it would suggest that the child is allergic to his own bacteria and that perhaps the use of bacterial vaccine will abort further attacks (see Chapter 8).

CUTS are most frequent in the two-year-old child who stumbles, falls, and opens a gash on his forehead. There is a good blood supply to the skin of the head, and the bleeding can be quite alarming. Basic steps are to clean the area with soap and water and apply a compression dressing to squash the blood vessels flat, thus controlling the bleeding. The next step is to determine whether the cut needs to be sutured. Surgeons like to suture things, so they will if you ask them, but doctors are finding that many cuts can be efficiently pulled together by taping. This is a satisfactory compromise, because cuts on the head heal rapidly. Besides, taping can be done with less physical and emotional trauma for the young child. In any event, some decision has to be made before six or eight hours have elasped. If the wound is left open after that time, infection can set in, and sometimes the wound *has* to be left open—which can mean scarring. It is routine to give a tetanus booster for any break in the skin, if the child has not received a booster within the previous twelve months.

When bleeding occurs, do not panic. Clean the wound; control bleeding with pressure and not a tourniquet; and make arrangements for medical help, whether it is suturing or taping.

FEVERS in children are most often due to virus infections that are self-limited, not serious, and untreatable by present-day medicine. For a child with fever, two rules of thumb are:

1. Give the child aspirin—one grain for every ten pounds of body weight, given every four hours. It takes an hour and a half for a dose to be effective. If the fever is reduced by a degree or two an hour and a half after administration, it implies the disease causing the fever is not serious.

2. The fever should not last for more than seventy-two hours. If it can be controlled with aspirin, and the child can take some nourishment and move about during the three days of fever, it implies that the child is controlling the infection and/or it is not serious and/or it is a virus.

FOREIGN OBJECTS such as beans, thumbtacks, erasers, and various other things are often inserted by small children in their noses and ears. Children with hay fever and a nasal itch often put wads of paper, raisins, or pills up their nostrils. These things frequently get lost up there and are difficult to get hold of. Many parents go after them with tweezers, but this only irritates the already inflamed nose. A trick I learned from an older doctor is to pinch shut the unaffected nostril and to blow sharply into the patient's mouth. The air pressure goes behind the nasal passage and pushes out the foreign object from inside. In effect, you blow the child's nose for him. Obviously, a tissue over the nose would keep you from getting the now-slimy object square in your face.

If a child has *swallowed* his foreign object, it is worth remembering that the narrowest passage is between the mouth and the stomach. If he is able to eat a piece of bread or a teaspoon of applesauce on top of his marble or keychain, it implies that the shiny little thing has at least reached his stomach. From there on, the rest of the journey is fairly simple. Occasionally a foreign object will get hung up at the anal sphincter, and sometimes has to be teased out with a lubricated finger. Pennies and dimes seem to travel through easily. A nickel possibly could get hung up, and a quarter almost always does. For some reason, sharp objects such as thumbtacks and pins almost never penetrate the intestinal wall en route through the body. It seems to recoil from the sharp object, which will tumble on through, possibly to get stuck at the anal opening.

Foreign objects in the ears sometimes have to be washed out with a syringe, and occasionally a nose-and-throat doctor has to use specially devised forceps to retrieve them. Objects that are inhaled are a special problem for the doctor who, under suitable anesthesia, has to go down into the bronchial tubing. Sudden onset of wheezing, coughing, turning blue, and gasping would usually give away the aspiration of a foreign object into the lung.

FROSTBITE was formerly treated by rubbing with ice or snow. It is now felt that the affected part—usually the fingers or toes—should be plunged into fairly hot water (105° to 110° F.). Even though there may be some pain, this system seems to unfreeze the part more rapidly than any other method and sometimes prevents the onset of gangrene, which can occur if the skin cells are frozen for any length of time.

HEAD INJURIES usually cause some concussion. Concussion is a swelling of the brain, the symptoms of which are headache, drowsiness, and vomiting. The skull may or may not be cracked; X rays of the skull are not as important as the symptoms. The pupils may or may not be dilated, constricted, or unequal. Concussion in most cases lasts six to ten hours, after which the victim's symptoms improve. If after twelve to twenty-four hours the headache, drowsiness, and vomiting become worse, then bleeding into or over the surface of the brain must be considered. It is not necessary to keep the patient awake in the first few hours to observe symptoms; it is probably better to allow him to sleep, but to arouse him every twenty to thirty minutes to evaluate his level of consciousness.

HEMORRHAGE means loss of blood, and should be controlled as soon as possible. The usual nasal hemorrhage or epistaxis is discussed under "Nosebleed." Look under "Cuts" for the treatment of skin cuts. Internal hemorrhage from the intestinal tract shows up as black, tarry, frequent stools. This would imply the ulceration of some area between the mouth and the lower bowel tract. Bright red blood found in the stools of small babies is quite common, and usually means that the stool has fissured the anal ring—a membrane that many babies have just inside the anal opening. This is not serious if it is spotty bleeding on the surface of the stool. Usually it is solved by gently prodding some petroleum jelly into the anal opening after each bowel movement, to grease the skids.

Bleeding from the ear after a head injury implies a skull fracture, and is a serious sign. It can also occur if a child has poked something into his ear, and the doctor should be consulted to make sure there is no permanent damage to the eardrum.

Blood in the urine can result from any one of twenty different causes. The most common one in a boy is an ulceration, usually the result of ammonia formation, just inside the opening of his penis. Passage of the salt urine over the ulceration, will cause the leakage of a little blood. It is not serious, and usually responds to the application of a bit of antibiotic ointment to the opening. A very effective way to get the ointment in the right place is to use an eye ointment, the tube of which has a pointed end and is just the right size for squirting a dollop of this ointment just inside. Obviously, the formation of ammonia also has to be controlled. If there is blood throughout the entire urinary stream, this implies bleeding from the kidneys and/or the bladder. Passage of dark brown or smoky urine suggest that the patient has Bright's disease or glomerulonephritis.

NOSE INJURY is common after falling face down or not catching a ball. It is actually difficult to break a small child's nose because of the large amount of cartilage that constitutes his nasal structure. If the nose has been struck and bleeds from the inside, it implies that the cartilage or bone has broken through the mucus membranes. Whether the bones are still in good alignment or not is difficult to tell. X rays may be necessary to determine this. In general, if the tip of the nose is centered between the pupils of the eyes when the patient is evaluated from the front view, then his nose may not be broken. Also, if the bridge of the nose is not depressed it may not be broken. However, many nose injuries result in a collection of old blood on one side or the other. This influences healing and stimulates one side of the nose to grow faster than the other. The patient may develop a deviated septum later in life, even though he might not have actually broken his nose.

It is difficult to know exactly what to do with a nose injury. If there is doubt, careful X rays will determine if bone segments are out of place. In the first twenty-four to forty-eight hours, these bones can be moved back to the proper position for healing. Otherwise—if they heal in incorrect positions—remedial surgery will be necessary later in life.

NOSEBLEEDS are common in children during cold, dry weather, during the hot summer, or after slight trauma. Old tricks like placing a cold knife on the back of the neck or putting ice on the lip or gums are of doubtful value. Almost all nosebleeds originate from eroded capillaries on the first one inch of the nasal septum. Pressure must be applied *there* to flatten the capillaries. Make a tampon by wetting a piece of tissue or part of a cotton ball; it should be big enough to just slide into the nostril. Sometimes a lubricant will help; some favor putting a few drops of a nose-drop solution on the surface of the wad to act as a vasoconstrictor. Push this into the nose and then pinch the wings of the nose together snugly for ten minutes. This should stop the bleeding. Leave the tampon in place for another ten minutes and then s-l-o-w-l-y withdraw it. This should leave a clear, open passageway free of clot. If a clot is allowed to form in the nose, it dries, cracks, and opens the vessels again. Some lubricant should be applied to the raw area for a week until healing is complete. If hemorrhage is frequent, cauterizing with a silver-nitrate stick may help.

POISONINGS usually demand induction of vomiting by giving syrup of ipecac. (It would be wise to have this in the house for emergencies.) If an overdose of aspirin, iron, tranquilizers, sedatives, etc. is ingested by a child, he should take three tea-spoons of the syrup. If he has not vomited by fifteen to twenty minutes, his stomach should be pumped. Some doctors recommend an emetic injection (apomorphine) which is efficient. Aspirin is still the most common poison that children get hold of, but this problem is being reduced because, by law, baby aspirin is now sold only in bottles containing about thirty tablets.

Most authorities now feel that if gasoline, kerosene, paint thinner, and related petroleum hydrocarbons are ingested, the child should *not* vomit. When he is retching, he may aspirate some of the material into his lungs. This causes a chemical type of pneumonia, which is more serious than leaving the particular hydrocarbon in the intestinal tract. Mineral oil might be advised.

When in doubt, call your doctor immediately (A poison control center is available in most large cities.)

Section II

DISEASES

ABSCESSES have four qualities: pain, redness, swelling, and heat (localized fever), all concentrated in one area. If the abscess is superficial (near the surface of the skin), hot packs are considered standard treatment. One method of packing an abcess involves three layers—first comes a hot, wet, salty one made from about a teaspoon of table salt or Epsom salt in a quart of hot water. A washcloth or Turkish towel is immersed in this solution and then wrung out and placed over the abscess. Completely enclosing this should be a plastic sheet to hold in the heat and moisture. Around this and extending beyond the edges of the plastic should be a big, dry bath towel or beach towel.

The hot pack is usually left on for twenty-four hours, at the end of which time the four abscess symptoms should be considerably reduced. After this, intermittent hot packing should be continued until the abscess localizes, points, and drains; or until the surgeon opens it, or until the body absorbs it. Your doctor, of course, may want to prescribe internal antibiotics; but moist, salty heat can be curative all by itself. If somebody suffers from repeated pustules, pimples, abscesses, and boils, it may mean that he is suffering from staphylococcus bacteria which he may be harboring in his nose. A suitable antibiotic cream is sometimes effective, if placed in the victim's nose twice a day for two weeks to break the vicious cycle.

Some people have had luck with injections of staphylococcus toxoid that may increase their immunity to the staphylococcus that produces most boils.

ATHLETE'S FOOT is a fungus infection which usually involves the webbing between the toes. This irritating condition can be found in any area that's dark and often moist, two conditions which promote the growth of fungus. Many people assume that any itchy, irritating, scaly condition of the feet is athlete's foot, but, if the rash is on either top or bottom surface of the foot, it is more likely to be a contact rash due to nylon in the stockings or plastic inserts in the shoes. The obvious way to control the latter condition is to wear white cotton stockings and leather shoes, or to go barefoot. For the athlete's foot fungus a new ointment is quite effective.

BRONCHITIS is an infection of the bronchial tubes, usually of bacterial origin. The victim has a hard cough and may raise purulent material. It tends to be triggered by a cold and requires some antibiotic for its cure. An abnormal number of bronchial infections—especially if each one is accompanied by an audible expiratory wheeze—suggests an allergy in the background. Most often it is an inhalation allergy, but it can be related to milk drinking and/or an allergy to the person's own bacteria. Appropriate measures are necessary to cut down the frequency of these attacks, because a bad bronchitis attack decreases the amount of oxygen that is getting to the brain, with resultant brain injury (see Chapter 8).

CAT SCRATCH disease is not uncommon. Apparently cats harbor the virus in their claws. An insignificant scratch can cause regional lymph nodes to swell alarmingly and even become big enough to break down and fester. There is no specific treatment, and the condition may drag on for some weeks. This is one of the disadvantages to having furry pets in the house, along with the possibility of the child developing an allergy to the animals. (Another disadvantage is that the mother is usually the one who must care for them.)

CELIAC DISEASE is a condition of chronic diarrhea, most commonly due to the intestines' inability to digest the glutins found in wheat products. It is not strictly an allergy, but acts like one. When the child eats flour products, he has a rather alarming amount of bloat and diarrhea. This condition is not to be confused with cystic fibrosis.

CHICKEN POX is the second most contagious disease in the world, the first being smallpox. Accordingly, it is usually contracted by a child before he is five or six. This is fortunate, because chicken pox is a very severe illness in an adult, and the complications are much more frequent. Also, the second case of chicken pox in a home is usually more violent than the first. Most doctors now believe that if an older child brings this disease home when there is a baby in the house, an injection of gamma globulin for the baby will make the disease lighter and the complications—such as high fever, pneumonia, or encephalitis—less likely. A significant number of victims get distressing sores in the mouth and down the throat. This symptom is usually associated with a high fever and general misery. Baking-soda baths and various lotions to pat on the skin are worth trying. At present, there are specific antihistaminics that help cut down on some of the itching.

Obviously, the more the child digs at his sores, the more likely is he to scar. However, I have seen some children who did not touch their skin and still had permanent pits, and others who scratched their skin unmercifully but did not develop scars. Doctors are trying to get the schools to change the laws about chicken pox, so that a child who is not too sick can come to school and expose the whole class. Then the majority of the population would be able to get it while they are still young. A child with uncomplicated chickenpox does not need to be confined to his bed and may be up and around the house—even outside. However, he is still contagious. Some doctors feel the possibility of contagion exists as long as there are sores on the skin, but most now feel that this is not true, and that probably no one is contagious once his pox (the water blisters) have dried up.

COMMON COLDS are virus infections that last seven days. In a baby there is usually some fever the first day or so, and the discharge from his nose is clear and watery. Often some sneezing accompanies the first day or two of a cold. About one out of three colds is triggered by an allergy. The use of antihistamines at the very first sniffle can abort some of these colds. If it lasts longer than a week, it is by definition not a cold: It is either an allergy or a secondary infection, in which case the secretions become green or yellow (see "Rhinitis").

CYSTITIS is a bladder infection. The victim usually has no fever but only burning, urgent, and frequent urination. A urinalysis reveals the presence of innumerable pus (or white) cells. Because the bacteria are usually the ones found in the colon, and because girls are much more likely to be affected, it is assumed that the responsible bacteria migrate up the urethra from the anal area. It is appropriate to teach girls to wipe themselves from the front to the rear after urination or defecation. Occasionally this condition is encouraged by an allergy and/or alkaline urine. If structural anomalies are ruled out as a cause, the diet should exclude milk and citrus drinks. Apple and cranberry juice acidify the urine and discourage bacteria growth.

DIARRHEA is the passage of frequent, watery stools. It usually is due to a virus, and in a child it almost always lasts seven days, as does a cold. Adults get over it more rapidly because they have more immunity, and often call it the "twelve-hour" or "twenty-four hour" flu.

Usually the victim starts with vomiting and ends up with diarrhea; there are usually intermittent cramps around the navel, accompanied by sunken eyes, paleness, and listlessness. The diet should be low in roughage consisting mainly of fluids. If there is no vomiting, milk may be added, followed by applesauce, bananas, and rice. If the stools have an especially offensive putrid odor, are bloody and the victim has a fever it may be one of the more severe varieties called dysentery (usually due to bacteria). There are appropriate medicines for this.

If the diarrhea seems to be due to the intestinal flu virus, but the watery stools last longer than a week, then several other considerations have to be taken into account: (1) the flu has stirred up an allergy to something that was safe to eat before, such as milk or wheat, (2) it is a secondary infection and should respond to appropriate antibiotics, (3) the patient is possibly deficient in some intestinal enzyme that breaks down sugars (if these enzymes are missing, the sugars ferment to cause diarrhea, gas, and bloat).

DIPHTHERIA is a severe disease manifested by a very painful sore throat and toxicity. Its poison can damage the heart and brain. It is a rare disease today because of the almost universal use of DPT shots.

ENCEPHALITIS is a general term for any inflammation of the brain —usually caused by virus infections and occasionally by mumps. Encephalitis can also be a complication of chicken pox or measles, but there are other, more rare forms. The usual symptoms are excruciating headache, fever, and sometimes a stiff neck and back. It can occur with polio, or be confused with meningitis, which is usually a bacterial infection. Bacterial meningitis can be treated with antibiotics, but encephalitis is almost always a varus and hence, untreatable. The dangers of encephalitis are its severe effects on the nervous system and the possibility of brain damage. Swelling of the brain may lead to coma. Cardiac and respiratory arrest may follow.

FLU is a general term for almost all virus infections. There is no specific medicine to combat viruses. The usual flu is an intestinal infection characterized by twenty-four hours of vomiting and seven days of diarrhea. The problem with this disease is that it can lead to dehydration from lack of fluid in the tissues. The virus called respiratory flu, or influenza, usually runs in winter epidemics. It is characterized by headache and fever for two or three days, and a strangling cough that lasts a week to ten days. Sometimes secondary complications can be treated with antibiotics.

FUNGUS INFECTIONS are common in children. The usual one we see is the scaly, slightly pinkish patch that occurs on the arms, neck, cheek, or shins of a child who has been in contact with an infected cat or dog. This type is usually treated with surface antifungus ointments. There is also a human type of fungus infection that affects the hair shafts in children who have picked it up from resting on infected furniture. Usually there is a bald circle on the scalp with a slight stubble growth. Antifungus medicines taken internally are almost always curative, but the results are not obvious for about six weeks. Athlete's foot is another fungus infection and usually produces cracked, itchy, tender skin in the webs between the toes. Surface antifungus ointments are usually curative.

GLOMERULONEPHRITIS is a kidney inflamation that follows an infection caused by a certain type of streptococcus. The patient usually passes bloody, brown urine and develops anemia, puffy lids, and hypertension. Penicillin is necessary. 80 percent of those afflicted recover, apparently completely, but some continue on to nephrosis, a condition of chronic fluid accumulation; cortisone drugs may be indicated.

HEMOPHILIA is a bleeding disease that affects males but is carried by females. There are many forms of hemophilia, depending on which part of the clotting complex is affected. The classical kind requires constant supervision, the avoidance of trauma, and often intravenous injections of antihemophiliac globulin and fresh blood.

HEPATITIS is an inflammation of the liver. There are now two recognized forms, both due to viruses. One is assumed to be contagious, and fairly common, usually manifesting itself by a dull aching in the upper right side of the abdomen, lethargy, and jaundice. The other type is called *serum hepatitis* and is usually transmitted intravenously. It can be a serious illness leading to malfunction of the liver over a long period. Occasional patients develop cirrhosis. If the first type of hepatitis shows up in a family, the rest of the members of the family are usually protected by the intramuscular use of gamma globulin.

HERPES is the general term for a virus inflammation, usually characterized by blisters that may occur on the mouth, the eyes, or the genitals. Some forms of herpes cause encephalitis; others are considered to be the source of adult shingles. Some doctors believe that the herpes virus lies dormant in people until triggered by the eating of certain foods such as chocolate, nuts, or citrus products. When exposed to the sun some patients develop herpes on their lips, while others seem to acquire them merely from emotional disturbances. Often those who have suffered repeatedly from herpes or canker sores have found that several vaccinations with smallpox vaccine will build up their immunity against further attacks.

IMPETIGO is a skin infection usually due to streptococcus or staphylococcus. Many ointments are very effective. The usual case is that of a child who has skinned his elbow or knee and has scratched at the wound, thereby introducing the infection. Impetigo is usually an oozy, crusty sore that can spread from one area of the body to another. An occasional child develops impetigo around his mouth after he eats such foods as chocolate or citrus products. These create a little rash or crack, and because he digs at it, a secondary infection develops. Ointments that can be purchased over the counter are effective, but in an extensive case it would be worthwhile to consult a physician about the use of internal antibiotics.

INFECTIOUS MONONUCLEOSIS is a virus infection; how it spreads is not completely clear; it used to be called the "kissing disease." It is most commonly seen in young adults. It usually develops as a fever with headache, sore throat, and swollen glands which increase in severity over a two-week period; and goes on to lethargy, weakness, sometimes swollen liver, and in 50 percent of the cases, a swollen spleen. There is a blood test usually reliable in diagnosis. Some patients are completely over the signs of infection within a month, but many others go on feeling poorly for long afterward. It is often difficult to determine when the disease has finally burned itself out.

An occasional patient develops encephalitis from this virus. The very worst complication is the possible rupture of the spleen, which may occur if the spleen is enlarged below the margin of the ribs. If so, the patient should not participate in contact sports of any kind until the spleen is again of normal size.

INFLUENZA is a general term for a virus respiratory infection. Usually it starts with fever, headaches, and painful burning eyeballs and ends up with a strangling cough. It commonly lasts about a week to ten days; a longer bout implies there is some secondary infection, and only if this is true would antibiotics be effective. Intestinal flu in a child usually lasts seven days—one day of vomiting and then diarrhea. The real problem with the illness is dehydration. Severe vomiting can be controlled with the use of a rectal suppository containing a tranquilizer. This usually controls the vomiting and hence controls the dehydration (see "Diarrhea" and "Flu").

LEUKEMIA is a condition in which there is a derangement of the white blood cells, usually the lymphocytes. Just ten years ago it was universally fatal in from six to twelve months. However, new medicines have been devised to control this, and there are now a few patients with arrested cases who are still alive after three to five years of treatment. Some researchers now feel that leukemia is due to a virus, and when viruses can be controlled we may be able to cure leukemia.

MEASLES (see "Rubeola").

MENINGITIS is a bacterial infection of the surface lining of the brain. It is usually considered to be blood-borne. Bacteria are carried from the nose or throat to the brain, where they create a usually characteristic set of symptoms—high fever, coma, and a stiff neck and back. Upon examination, pus is found in the spinal fluid. Antibiotics, if given early enough, are usually curative, and if the infection is not too overwhelming, the patient can usually be saved. One type, due to the meningococcus, is considered to be contagious; the others, because the infection is quite well locked up inside the brain, are not.

The meningococcus type is often found in school dormitories or army or navy barracks where many people live together. It used to respond very nicely to sulfa drugs, but some strains are now becoming quite resistant. It is rapid, overwhelming, sudden in onset, and sometimes fatal before diagnosis can be made and treatment instituted.

MONILIA, or *thrush*, usually shows up as a superficial skin rash in the diaper area of a baby, or as white, milk-curd–like spots inside the mouth. It is assumed to come from the mother, who may be suffering from a thrush infection of the vagina. Newborns usually acquire it during the first two weeks of life, and it may spread to other parts of the body. In the diaper area, it is a very bright red, solid rash with a fairly sharply demarcated border. What look like pustules line the edge of the rash. There are new ointments that are curative, but a baby will get it again from his mother if her condition is not cured.

MUMPS (or Epidemic Parotitis) is a virus inflammation of the salivary glands. The victim is usually five to eight years old and acquires it from his classmates. Characteristically, he has swollen cheeks that fill out the pocket below the ear lobe—not to be confused with the swollen glands from tonsillitis, which are high in the neck under the corner of the jawbone. In general, this is not a serious infection unless it (1) leads to encephalitis, in which case the patient may be severely incapacitated with a high fever and an exquisite headache or (2) goes to the pan-

creas and produces a severe stomachache, fever, and vomiting.
There is now a live mumps vaccine that seems to give permanent protection from this disease. There is no medical reason why a patient with mumps cannot be ambulatory if he
feels well enough for it. He may select his own diet, but it is
true that sour foods such as pickles and lemons may give him
some jaw spasm.

ORCHITIS is an inflammation of the testicle; it is most commonly seen as a complication of mumps and it occurs only in
mature males (one out of four who get the mumps will develop orchitis). In about 20 percent of the cases, it will be bi-
lateral. There seems to be no positive correlation between
physical activity and the development of mumps orchitis.
Statistics indicate that patients who have been flat on their
backs in bed with mumps will develop this as frequently as
patients who have been up. Sometimes the pain is so distressing
that morphine is necessary. Surgery can help relieve the pressure.

OSTEOMYELITIS is an infection in the shaft of a bone. It is assumed
that a bacteria—usually staphylococcus—has been carried to the
area via the blood stream. A sudden high fever and pain usher
in the disease. Massive doses of appropriate antibiotics are
usually necessary for two to four weeks to prevent the bone
from being eaten away.

OTITIS is ear inflammation. External otitis is sometimes called
"swimmers' ear," and is an inflammation of the lining of the
ear canal, usually related to fungus or bacterial infection.
Otitis media is an inflammation just behind and on the eardrum. It is extremely painful and very common in children
getting over colds, although rare after the age of seven. If not
treated adequately, the infection can lead to deafness and mas-
toid inflammation. In patients who have been successfully
treated, a secretion sometimes is left behind the eardrum that
leads to deafness and that must be drained by aspiration. Repeated middle-ear infections are usually due to enlarged adenoids, but are sometimes a complication of nasal allergies. Tonsil and adenoid removal is often required to reduce the incidence.

PHARYNGITIS is another name for sore throat, and if tonsils are present, they are usually involved as well. Over 50 percent of sore throats are due to a streptococcus; others are due to viruses or other bacteria. Streptococcal pharyngitis (or tonsillitis) is the one form that should be diagnosed and treated. Penicillin is the appropriate remedy, but erythromycin is used if the patient is truly allergic to penicillin. It is important that treatment be continued for ten days to prevent the possibility of rheumatic involvement or kidney inflammation. Most doctors try to culture the throat to determine if the germ is the *hemolytic streptococcus*—the one most likely to lead to rheumatic fever.

PITYRIASIS ROSEA is a fairly common skin infection that dermatologists now think is due to a virus. There is usually a "herald" spot that looks like a skin fungus or ringworm. Within two weeks, the patient will notice fawn-colored, scaly, oval lesions over his trunk that may or may not itch. (It almost never occurs on the arms and legs.) Pityriasis lasts about a month and is usually considered noncontagious.

PNEUMONIA is a lung infection that can be caused by a variety of organisms. The old-fashioned lobar pneumonia is due to the pneumococcus, and is almost always susceptible to penicillin. Patients can have bronchial pneumonia in which patches of infected lung area are seen as spots on an X-ray. The treatment is usually the same. There is also a type of virus pneumonia that is difficult to treat except by certain antibiotics, a high fever, cough, and occasionally bloody sputum are the usual signs. If the pneumonia infection is close to the rib cage, it can give chest pain called *pleurisy*.

POLIOMYELITIS is a virus infection rarely seen these days because of the almost universal use of Salk or Sabin vaccine. The three types of polio all lead to similar symptoms: nerve inflammation creating a stiff neck and headache, and eventually, paralysis of certain muscle groups in a high percentage of the patients.

PYELITIS is a bacterial infection of the kidney. The female is more commonly affected. The onset is often sudden, accompanied by chills, fever, and backache. Antibiotics are usually necessary for one to three weeks. Repeated attacks suggest some anatomical defect in the tubing (ureters) leading from the kidneys to the bladder.

PYLORIC STENOSIS is a hypertrophy of the muscles at the outlet of the stomach leading to the duodenum. It is almost universally seen in the firstborn male child, frequently in the springtime. The child may be perfectly well until he is two or three weeks old, and then begin to vomit, often projectilely. His stools become firmer and less frequent, and he loses weight and suffers from dehydration and malnutrition. An operation is curative. There is a tendency for this condition to occur in families.

RABIES is an almost universally fatal disease, fortunately rare in our country. Dogs, once considered to be the prime carriers, are now rarely afflicted. Foxes, bats, and skunks are more likely to carry the illness, although the bite of most rodents is not usually a mode of transmission. Experts are unsure whether the rabies treatment is actually effective, or whether the patient getting the treatment would not have contracted the illness in the first place. But until better methods are found to determine whether the patient is going to develop rabies or not, the only recourse is to give him the series of injections.

RHEUMATIC FEVER occurs in 3 to 5 percent of those who have had an untreated streptococcal infection. It usually affects the heart valves and produces swollen, tender joints. At present, anybody who suffers rheumatic fever should be on continuous (and perhaps permanent) prophylactic treatment with penicillin or a related drug.

RHINITIS is the inflammation of the nose, sometimes called the common cold. The secretion is a watery discharge, and there may be fever and sneezing. If the discharge is clear, watery, or milky, it is considered a virus. The rhinitis virus usually lasts a week in a child and occasionally makes him susceptible to secondary infections such as bronchitis or otitis media. If the secretions become green or yellow, it indicates an upper respiratory bacterial infection or a purulent rhinitis, which are treatable.

If the watery, runny nose lasts longer than a week, nasal allergy has to be considered. In this case, the victim usually notices a stinging, burning, itching sensation in his nose. If it occurs only in the springtime, it is usually due to pollens; if only when the child is in bed, a feather pillow or wool blanket is usually responsible. Occasionally people will suffer when they are near cats or dogs to which they are sensitive. Antihistamines will sometimes control rhinitis symptoms even if due to a virus. In babies, nose drops are often used to clear the nasal passages, but it is recommended that they be used two or three times a day for only three or four days, and then be discontinued for a day or two. Some children can get sensitive to nose drops, which will then do them more harm than good (see "Common cold").

RINGWORM (see "Fungus infections").

ROSEOLA occurs in a baby somewhere between the age of six months and two years, often when he is cutting teeth. It is a virus infection believed to be one of the measles, usually characterized by seventy-two hours of a high fever, often 105° or 106° F. Aspirin almost always controls the fever temporarily, and when it subsides, the patient breaks out in a usually flat, red rash on his stomach, back, and face. The rash almost never appears on arms and legs. Roseola is not contagious and usually has no complications, although some babies develop a convulsion when the fever occurs.

RUBELLA is German or three-day measles. In a child the fever rarely goes over 100° F. The rash appears suddenly, all over on the first day, and each individual spot is not over one-fourth of an inch in diameter. The giveaways of this illness are its mildness and the swollen, somewhat tender lymph glands found just behind the ears. It is now well-documented that a woman one or two months pregnant who develops Rubella has a 20 to 40 percent chance of producing a baby with cataracts, deafness, heart lesions, or mental deficiency. It is not known positively whether a large dose of gamma globulin will prevent the exposed pregnant woman from developing this disease or help modify its damaging effects on the baby. Any woman who develops German measles in the first two months of pregnancy should seriously consider these risks and consult her doctor.

RUBEOLA is another name for the hard, coughing, black or two-week measles. There are harmful effects from this illness, so every one-year-old should be given the live measles vaccine, which is 98 percent effective in preventing the illness. Because of the common use of the vaccine, this disease is rapidly disappearing. If a child is not vaccinated and has been exposed to rubeola, he should be given a shot of gamma globulin to ward off the disease. A high percentage of victims will develop hearing difficulties or behavior problems as a result of inflammation in the brain. The adverse effects of light during the measles is an old wives' tale. With all measles, the eyes become light-sensitive, but the virus rather than the light is responsible for any vision damage.

SCABIES is a skin inflammation due to the burrowing of the female mite, which lays its eggs in little tunnels just below the surface of the skin. Scabies is usually found in the pulse side of the wrist, in warm places near the armpit, and in the groin. It is sometimes called the seven-year itch, but new ointments are effective in killing the egg-laying mother. Since insects travel, scabies is contagious.

SCARLATINA is another form of strep sore throat, but in this case the rash is more spotted and appears mainly on the warm places around the armpits and groin. The treatment is the same as for strep sore throat or scarlet fever.

SCARLET FEVER is a sore throat due to a certain type of streptococcus that produces circumoral pallor (no rash about mouth) and an extensive, continuous red rash over most of the body. It is dangerous only to the extent that if untreated, this particular streptococcus is more likely to lead to rheumatic fever. Penicillin or a related drug is the best remedy and should be continued for ten days. Authorities disagree as to whether everybody in the house should be given prophylactic medication to help them avoid the illness.

SINUSITIS is a bacterial infection in which a sinus becomes congested with pus. It is usually secondary to an inhalation allergy, cold, or structural defect which blocks the sinus opening to the nasal cavity. Pus backs up, fills the sinus cavity, and results in fever and pain.

SMALLPOX is uncommon at the present time in our country, due to the almost universal use of smallpox vaccination. It is en-

demic in certain parts of Africa and Asia, and the death rate
is one out of two. New treatments have been developed for
this condition, but because so few American doctors have seen
smallpox, diagnosis is often delayed until too late. The first
smallpox vaccination should be at or after the first birthday.
If it is given earlier, the complications are sometimes severe.
The smallpox vaccination should never be given to a child
with eczema, or if there is a child in the house who has eczema
or any other skin infection.

STAPHYLOCOCCUS infections are fairly common and very difficult
to eradicate, since the staphylococcus germ has become resistant to many antibiotics. Usually staphylococcus is found in
people who suffer from sties, boils, abscesses, furuncles, and
the paronychia or the "run-around" that develops around
fingernails. It can be a family disease, and sometimes heroic
measures are necessary to rid a house of this infection. It is
thought that anybody who has been in a hospital may carry
the staphylococcus infection home with him on his nasal mu-
cosa. (This is less true today because of better control methods.) Occasionally, spread of the infection can be interrupted
by placing antibiotic ointment in the victim's nose, or by in-
jecting a staphylococcus toxoid vaccine.

STIES are painful, red swellings in the eyelid, usually due to the
staphylococcus that forms a small pimple or boil in one of the
hair follicles. It finally gets big enough and drains pus and
blood, but the germs from this lesion can reinfect other areas
of the eyelid. It is discussed under "Staphylococcus."

STOMATITIS is an inflammation of the mouth, sometimes confused
with hoof-and-mouth disease, or trench mouth. It is usually
due to a virus. Characteristic inflammation is seen during the
summer in a two-year-old child who develops a high fever
and a number of canker sores in and around his mouth. The
child will sit and cry with his mouth open, and will let the
saliva run out of his mouth because it is too painful to swallow.
The fever lasts seventy-two hours or so, but the sores take a
week to heal.

STREPTOCOCCUS is a bacteria, usually leading to streptococcal sore
throat and frequently found in skin infections such as impetigo.

STRIDOR is noisy breathing often seen in the newborn baby. It does not interfere with his eating and sleeping, but it may last for several months, and produces noises that can alarm the parents who have to listen. It is generally considered due to relaxed vocal cords that flop back and forth. The condition takes care of itself when the vocal cords eventually firm up. Occasionally it comes from extra mucus in the throat and can be related to a milk allergy.

TETANUS is a serious, often fatal disease, but is almost never seen in properly immunized people. One form of newborn tetany occurs when a baby delivered at home has his umbilical cord tied by an unsterile shoelace. The DPT baby shots contain immunizing material against tetanus. Shots are usually repeated at eighteen months or two years, and again prior to school. After this time, diphtheria and tetanus shots are given on a routine basis every ten years, but a booster is usually considered necessary if the patient suffers a puncture wound or break in the skin when more than a year has elapsed since the last shot.

THRUSH (see "Monilia").

TONSILLITIS is an inflammation of the tonsils. Well over half the cases are due to streptococcus bacteria. Occasionally what looks like a classical streptococcus tonsillitis can be due to a virus, and is a self-limiting disease requiring no treatment. In most tonsillitis cases it is probably worthwhile to take a throat culture and determine whether streptococcus is involved. Because of the possibility of trouble with rheumatic fever, it is important that treatment be continued for ten days following certain types of streptococcus infection. Tonsils are usually somewhat enlarged from age four to six, but after age seven they usually shrink up and are an infrequent cause of trouble. If tonsillitis occurs more than two or three times a year after age seven, it is worth considering a tonsillectomy.

TUBERCULOSIS is slowly disappearing from our country, but not really fast enough. Routine skin testing for TB should be done every two to three years in the growing child. If the skin test is positive, it is assumed that the child has been exposed to an open case of tuberculosis some time since the last negative skin test, and all his contacts should be tested. Primary tuberculosis is not considered contagious, but should be treated to reduce the chance of spread and cavity formation. About one out of every two adults have positive skin tests to tuberculosis, implying that they have been exposed to the bacteria but did not develop the active, full-blown disease. It is important that teachers, food-handlers, and others in contact with children be routinely screened by skin test or chest X ray.

TYPHOID FEVER in our country is becoming less common with modern sanitary practices. The few outbreaks are almost always traceable to some carrier or "Typhoid Mary" who does not display symptoms. The disease is usually manifested by a high fever and terrible diarrhea which may lead to the ulceration of the intestinal tract and severe dehydration. New antibiotics usually cure this condition.

VARICELLA (see "Chickenpox").

VIRUS is a term used to designate a growing particle that lives inside the cell. It is the usual cause of various types of flu and most of the childhood contagious diseases such as mumps, chicken pox, and measles; and possibly other conditions such as warts and pityriasis, and even cancer and leukemia. There are no satisfactory medicines for viruses at the present time. Because viruses do not live outside the body, close contact with infected individuals is the only means of spread.

WHOOPING COUGH in infancy is a dread disease because of the severe malnutrition and coughing paroxysms that can lead to cyanosis in small babies. It is rare to find this disease in a properly immunized child. Although immunization does not necessarily prevent someone from getting whooping cough, the case is usually much milder. Although it is a bacterial infection, whooping cough responds poorly to antibiotics. There is a whooping cough immune serum globulin that is fairly effective in controlling the severity and the extent of the disease. Other diseases due to related bacteria have symptoms similar to whooping cough.

Section III

CONDITIONS AND
DEFINITIONS

ABDOMEN It is worthwhile to know the various areas of the abdomen, so that when consulting your doctor, you will be able to communicate more effectively.

The right upper section is associated with the liver and gall bladder.

The mid-upper area (the soft section just below the sternum or breastbone) is the stomach area, usually where ulcer pains are located.

The upper left area overlies the spleen—a lump or swelling in this area might conceivably indicate an enlarged spleen and/or kidney.

The right mid-flank is where one finds the right kidney and the ascending colon.

The periumbilical or midsection is where most stomach cramps originate. This is the pain most often felt with vomiting and diarrhea. Crampy pains that come and go can be due to an obstruction, but are usually traceable to intestinal flu.

The left mid-flank and lower left area are involved with the descending colon and large colon; pain there might indicate constipation, pinworms, or trouble with the left kidney.

The lower right section is the usual site of the appendix.

In the lower mid-area are located the bladder and, in females, the uterus.

ACETONE is found in abnormally high quantities in the blood and urine of patients with inadequate carbohydrate metabolism. Acetone is also found in the urine when body fats are being utilized as fuel—as during periods of vomiting, starvation, diarrhea, and fever.

ACHONDROPLASIA is a genetic form of dwarfism, due to a cartilage growth deficiency that mainly afflicts the long bones of the arms and legs. The head and trunk are of almost normal proportion.

ACIDOSIS occurs when the body loses enough alkali substances to shift its Ph balance to the acid side. It is common in children with diarrhea and diabetes (which cause a loss of sodium), aspirin poisoning (which accumulates acetylsalicylic acid), and kidney disease (which causes losses of alkali or other bases). Blood tests can accurately diagnose the severity of the derangement and suggest what replacement therapy is needed. Moderate to severe cases usually require intravenous infusions of alkali-rich solutions.

ACNE brands some 60 to 80 percent of all adolescents. One very severe kind causes deep pustules and sometimes disfiguring boils that lead to scarring. This type of acne needs the almost constant attention of your doctor and/or skin specialist.

There are some routine things that adolescents should know about this usually mild skin condition. One of the most important remedies is cleanliness. Soap and water used with a clean washcloth is the most effective treatment, but it is not a cure; it will only control the spread of infection to other pores. Diet aggravates the condition in many cases, and cola drinks and chocolate are almost taboo. Milk (with its fatty deposits) can often aggravate acne, and skim milk might be a wise choice for the milk-drinking adolescent. Some complexions have benefited from carefully measured doses of exposure to sunshine or a sunlamp. Various applications help to dry the skin. Your druggist may be able to help you with medications that you can buy over the counter, but seek the advice of a doctor or skin specialist if these are ineffective.

ADDISON'S DISEASE is a rather rare condition due to injury or malfunction of the adrenal glands. The victim is weak, wasted, and pigmented; he may crave salt and water. The absent adrenal hormones can now be supplied artificially.

ADENOIDS, if enlarged, create nasal speech in most children. They ordinarily swell up from age three to six, but from age seven on they are supposed to slim down again, eliminating the nasal quality. The worst adenoids can do is to plug the eustachian tubes, whose openings are found at the sides of the adenoids. If this body of tissue is big enough to plug up the eustachian tubes, a fluid accumulates behind the eardrum, or at least retraction. Either of these conditions can lead to repeated ear infections and deafness. If a child develops chronic ear trouble, you should determine the advisability of having his adenoids removed. (Usually tonsils are removed at the same time.)

The farther away the trouble is from the adenoids and tonsils the less likely will their removal do any good. The victim of a chronic cough may find that his cough is worse as if the adenoids and tonsils were protecting his lungs from the infections in the upper respiratory tract, or if his cough was due to an allergy in the first place. Before contemplating an operation, allergies must be ruled out.

ADOPTION by definition, is the rearing of another's child as your own. Anxiety about continuing custody can best be avoided by following legal adoption processes through a recognized and reliable agency. Since hereditary and prenatal factors are often incompletely known, the baby should be given a thorough physical examination during the newborn period and before he is brought home from the hospital. Many adoptive parents would find it no hardship to care for a child who had a minor anomaly, but in any case, the parents should be aware of what to expect from the child and what is expected of them.

No one has been able to determine exactly when a child should be told of his adoptive status; the decision has to be made by the individual family. I assume any behavior or emotional problems in these children would be caused by a combination of inherited and environmental factors as is the case in any other home. The joys of filling a home with a human being to receive and give love are a great reward to many couples whose lives would be incomplete without parenthood.

ADRENALIN (see "Epinephrine").

ALBUMINURIA is the presence of albumin—protein—in the urine. Some is normal, but when amounts are large enough to be detected by the usual laboratory methods, it suggests kidney disease, most likely glomerulonephritis (which follows certain streptococcal infections). A benign form that is related to sitting or standing and disappears after lying down is called *orthostatic*.

ALLERGY, in general, is a sensitivity to something inhaled, eaten, or in contact with the skin. The more one looks for allergies, the more likely they are to be found. The usual allergy in children is rhinitis, or the watery, drippy nose. The associated itch forces the child to rub or pick his nose. Allergies can mask as other conditions and may even be the cause of headaches, stomachaches, or bed-wetting (see Chapter 8).

ALOPECIA is baldness. If a child has circular patches of stubble where his hair shafts have broken, you may suspect a fungus invasion. New oral medicine is rapidly curative. If you note irregularly shaped areas of complete hair loss, the condition is alopecia areata. Virus, emotion, injury, fever, or tight hair styles like the "pony tail" are also culprits. Hair usually grows back within six months without treatment.

AMBLYOPIA means blindness. It usually refers to a condition called suppression amblyopia, which is usually related to strabismus or crossed eyes. In this situation, the brain seems to be confused by the two visual images it receives from the eyes—in other words, double vision. The brain simply blocks out the image it gets from one eye. The victim will retain peripheral vision, but is unable to see things clearly and sharply. At age four his visual acuity may drop from 20-20 to 20-30 down to 20-400 or worse. If a child is cross-eyed and no attempt is made to correct the problem, amblyopia may set in. Something should be done before age three, since doctors are rarely able to treat it after age five.

AMEBIC DYSENTERY is characterized by bloody diarrhea. The condition is caused by a one-celled parasite in the colon, and is sometimes difficult to treat.

AMMONIACAL DIAPER usually occurs in the morning. The strong ammonia smell is due to bacterial action that changes the urea in the urine to ammonia. Some babies are terribly sensitive to ammonia and develop redness, blisters, and ulcers. Boiling and bleaching the diapers are of no benefit. Some attempt must be made to (1) destroy the bacteria that live in the diaper and (2) counteract the ammonia. The diapers can be soaked in various bacteriocidal solutions, or they can be put out in the sunshine. If there are no bacteria, then the ammonia will not form. Pouring an ounce of vinegar in the second of four night diapers will acidify the urine. Adding extra water to the child's diet will not wash the ammonia out and only serves to make the condition worse: The more urine produced, the more ammonia will form. You should make an effort to cut down the child's fluid intake. In general, if he is urinating two or three times a day, he is probably getting a sufficient amount of fluid.

AMPHETAMINE is the generic name for the drug Benzedrine, manufactured by Smith, Kline and French Company. This medicine is effective in lengthening the short attention span that some children have which interferes with academic performance (see Chapter 5).

ANEMIA means weak or thin blood. The most common cause is lack of iron. Anemias due to other factors are rare. The most common one seen in children is iron-deficiency anemia, largely due to the milk diet that the child has been on in the first year or so of life. Nowadays, some formula milks are supplied with enough iron to prevent this deficiency anemia. Many children get anemic even though they are on a good general diet of meat, fruit, grain, and vegetables. But a child is most likely to become anemic if he is growing rapidly and living mostly off milk, bread, carbohydrates, and other white foods. Even if he is on a good diet, he may occasionally need some iron tonic. After a blood test, the doctor would be the best one to decide how much iron should be given and for how long.

ANESTHESIA is any substance used to deaden pain sense. Each surgeon has his favorite chemical to provide patient cooperation. An adult might tolerate hypnosis, ice, or a local anesthesia for some minor procedure (wart removal, suturing, tonsillectomy, tooth repair) which would panic a child. Under ten years of age, general anesthesia is usually necessary for surgery. If possible, elective or corrective surgery is best delayed until the patient is old enough to understand and cooperate. Even though reassured, the child under four or five may be overly anxious because of his fear of the unknown. He may think he is being punished for something he has done, so it is better to delay surgery until over six.

ANOREXIA is the loss of appetite, most commonly noticed between the ages of two and four. The child usually gains two to five pounds a year and needs little food to maintain this rate of growth. When the two-and-a-half-year-old eats one poor meal a day, his mother thinks he will surely get sick if he does not eat more. The father is not much help because he forces the food down, and the child soon returns it in an unreusable form.

ANOXIA is a term often used to describe the lack of oxygen some children suffer either before, during, or after delivery; during a high fever and convulsion, or during a severe attack of pneumonia or bronchitis. The condition is usually manifested by cyanosis or blueness. Not all anoxia is permanently harmful, but it can lead to specific injuries to the nervous system. In general, the earlier in life and the longer the anoxia, the more danger of damage.

ANTIBIOTICS are medicines that are used to kill bacteria. However, 80 percent of the infections that we see in children are due to viruses, which are not affected by antibiotics. A possible exception is virus pneumonia, which may be a large enough virus to respond to some of the mycins.

Antibiotics should be reserved for reasonably severe infections, and are not to be used indiscriminately. It is not wise to administer antibiotics in an effort to ward off secondary bacterial infections. Often, they simply make the bacterial infection resistant to that antibiotic. The biggest disadvantage to antibiotics is that the patient may become allergic to them or develop diarrhea.

ANTIDOTE is a remedy, usually one that counteracts the effects of a poison. The so-called "universal antidote" contains carbon black that helps to absorb noxious substances in the stomach. Prevention is the best antidote, and you must carry out periodic inspection of lethal areas (medicine cabinet, cupboard under sink, garage) if you are sheltering an orally inquisitive child. Toddlers seem to feel they understand things better if they can taste and eat them, and their curiosity kills hundreds of them every year. Syrup of ipecac is an emetic and should be in every home for instant use.

ANTIHISTAMINES are used for the control and suppression of allergic conditions. They come in a variety of forms and sizes, and almost every drug company makes a few. They have proved especially helpful for hay-fever sufferers. If a child has a sniffle that can be relieved by antihistamines, our assumption is that this condition is an allergy. Some have found antihistamines helpful in suppressing motion sickness or encouraging a reluctant child to drop off to sleep. In this latter regard, they sometimes work better than barbiturates.

ANUS is the terminal opening of the intestinal tract. Since this area contains many nerve endings, it is sometimes the focus of all sorts of psychological and physical problems. A child who keeps digging and poking at his rectum is usually suffering from worms, although irritating substances in the diet, such as citrus fruits or peaches, may produce the same effect. A new baby may have a tight ring of tissue just inside his anal opening, with resulting colic. The wise mother pays as little attention to this area as is possible. Reasonable cleanliness is all that is necessary.

It is better to soften constipated stools with a high roughage diet. The overly conscientious mother may produce a child who becomes overly concerned about his bowel activities.

APPETITE is related to many things, among them parental attitudes, congenital factors, ability to absorb and digest food, state of the bowels, state of mind, age, and rate of growth. The wise mother can whet her child's appetite by offering nourishing meals pleasantly served in congenial, unhurried surroundings. Although a bad appetite does not imply ill health, a good appetite generally is, of course, a good sign. A *change* in appetite suggests a possible problem. If a child laughs and smiles more than half the time, and is up and moving around, he is probably getting enough to eat. Encouraging him to eat more will only make him fat or frustrated. (Some children will go hungry if they know it bothers their mothers.)

ARTIFICIAL RESPIRATION is best accomplished by mouth-to-mouth breathing. The idea is to inflate the lungs of the non-breathing, comatose patient so that enough oxygen can be transported to the blood stream to reach the brain—the organ first to suffer if deprived of oxygen. Occasionally, heart massage is necessary also, and everyone should be familiar with both techniques.

ASCORBIC ACID (see "Vitamin C").

ASPIRIN, a remedy for fever and pain, was discovered almost one hundred years ago. A few people are sensitive to the drug, but there are now some aspirin substitutes that work almost as well. A good rule to remember is: one grain of aspirin for every ten pounds of body weight; this amount can be safely given every four hours. Each dosage takes about an hour and a half to work. If the fever is reduced or the headache is better within an hour and a half, then the condition is probably not too serious.

It is wise not to have too much baby aspirin in the house. A dose of one grain for every pound could be dangerous. If a child has eaten more than this amount, you should make him vomit by giving him syrup of ipecac. If this is not available, his stomach should be pumped. Aspirin is an acid, and an overdose may sometimes put the body into a state of irreversible acidosis.

ASTHMA occurs when the bronchial tubes go into spasm, usually due to some allergy or infection. Asthma produces a characteristic wheeze on expiration, which can easily be detected by having the victim breathe into the observer's ear. The victim has considerably more trouble exhaling than inhaling. This is a reasonably serious condition, and you should follow the doctor's advice. In most children, asthma is usually triggered by some infection or an infection is superimposed on an inhalation allergy.

ATELECTASIS is the collapse of a portion of a lung, most frequently seen in the premature baby. It may also be associated with asthma or bronchitis. If extensive, the blood flowing through this collapsed segment will not be properly oxygenated and the victim will become blue. The lack of oxygen may be significant enough to hurt areas of the baby's brain, leading to the hypermotor syndrome.

AUTISM is a type of childhood schizophrenia or psychosis, chiefly characterized by inability to respond socially or emotionally.

The play of such a child is nonexistent, inappropriate, or infantile. Communication is completely disorganized; the victim
appears deaf or retarded. Improvement is possible, but treatment is prolonged and difficult.

BACTERIA are unicellular organisms that can cause a wide variety
of diseases, most of which are treatable with antibiotics. A few
examples: the *pneumococcus* causes lobar pneumonia, the
streptococcus scarlet fever. Both of these bacteria are rapidly
destroyed by penicillin. The typhoid bacterium can usually be
eradicated by *ampicillin*, a form of penicillin. But the *staphylococcus*, which frequently causes boils, has become somewhat
resistant to penicillin, and other drugs are needed.

BARBITURATES are a widely used group of drugs for the treatment of anxiety, insomnia, seizures, and other nervous disorders. They are cheap and relatively safe, but some patients
may become habituated to their use.

BASAL METABOLISM is the sum of all the work done by the cells
of the body in the resting state. Because oxygen is required
for cellular metabolism, the body's efficiency can be measured
by calibrating how much oxygen is utilized in a given period
of time. A breathing test was formerly used to discover
hypo- or hyper-thyroidism, but has been supplanted by blood
chemical tests.

BATHING, as people have learned over the centuries, not only
makes the individual socially acceptable, but prevents a number of skin infections. Bathing usually discourages the growth
of various small chiggers, mites, and lice that some of our
not-so-remote ancestors were prone to harbor on their person.
Most odors that people have are due to the growth of bacteria
and fungus, and putting on clean clothing after a bath seems
to help discourage them.

Most mothers are baffled when they are faced with bathing
their new baby. They feel that this must be done only by an
expert. Most hospitals have a nurse who demonstrates the
procedure as if it were almost a religious rite. As a matter of
fact, a baby's bath should be quick and simple, and pleasant
for everyone.

For a new baby, it is usually not necessary to do more than
go over his dirty, sweaty areas with a wet washcloth. When

he starts to sleep through the night, a full bath is necessary, or a somewhat disagreeable odor will develop. Neither is it necessary to postpone the whole immersion bath until the cord is completely healed. Actually, it might be better to bathe this raw area so that it will be cleaner and less likely to support dangerous bacteria. Most of us recommend the use of liquid soaps that contain hexachlorophene as the most satisfactory way of cleaning without too much irritation. Most soaps are alkaline, and alkaline-treated skin is more susceptible to rashes, drying, and cracking. Bathing your baby in a plastic dishpan is probably preferable to the hard sink. Make sure the water is pleasantly warm and use as little soap as possible. If your baby has a great deal of cradle cap or scaly scalp, it is worthwhile to rub in some mineral oil before the bath to soften the scales. Then soap and a soft brush may effectively remove the scaliness. Some oily material naturally found in the genitalia is protective, and vigorous effort to remove it is unwise. Dry thoroughly in the armpits and between the fingers and toes. Some doctors recommend using alcohol to clean the navel, but it is too drying; the navel often cracks and bleeds. It might be better to use petroleum jelly or antibiotic ointment in this area. Powders are not necessary. Powder is a severe irritant, and if a baby gets a sprinkling of this in his eyes or inhales some, he will be quite unhappy. Baby oils can produce a pleasant, perfumed odor on the baby—and often make him break out with a contact rash! If his skin is dry, and oil is necessary, a very small amount of mineral oil is the safest thing to put on the scaly areas. Bathtime is a pleasant time to stimulate, cuddle, sing, and tickle your baby—an opportunity to offer love and warmth.

BEHAVIOR The purpose of this whole book is to help mothers determine whether their child is more or less normal. I am of the opinion that two sets of factors determine behavior: (1) the potential, genetic, or inherited ones and (2) the environmental ones. Apparently normal children in apparently normal environments can have miserable personalities, and others in terrible environments can grow up to be reasonably adequate, nonneurotic adults. The worst results would follow when a child with some nervous instability is reared in an unloving environment. Early diagnosis of abnormal behavior is mandatory; the old saw of "he will outgrow it" almost never applies. Children with peculiar behavior usually become terribly disturbed in adolescence, when many pressures from their hormones and from their environments cause unfavorable clashes. Preventive behavior modification in the early years is a more satisfactory approach.

BELL'S PALSY is a weakness or paralysis of the muscles on one side of the face, due to a malfunctioning of the facial nerve. The nerve passes near the middle ear and may have been hurt or injured by an ear infection or by forceps pressure at birth.

BIOPSY is the piece of tissue removed, usually in surgery, for closer inspection under a microscope. This examination aids in the diagnosis of a diseased organ when palpation or inspection are inadequate. For example, a small piece of a breast lump is often removed so that the pathologist can determine if cancer is present in a frozen section of the tissue. He can then rapidly signal the waiting surgeon, and a decision can be made regarding radical breast removal.

BIRTH, the first violent crisis you and your child have to face, should be as nontraumatic as possible. We know that women under eighteen and women over thirty-five have a much greater chance of both pregnancy and birth anomalies. An obstetrician can control many of the factors of abnormal birth, but, of course, a certain amount of chance and luck are involved on that fateful day. You should have complete trust and reliance in your obstetrician, because he can help you better than anyone else. The biggest problem to avoid is the anoxia, hypoxia, or lack of oxygen to the nervous system; this cannot help but do a certain amount of damage to the baby. The doctor usually does not use too much anesthesia on the mother, so that her baby will be able to initiate respiration himself and not be too dopey. If the doctor does not happen to be in time, nurses will usually allow delivery to proceed if it seems normal. In some cases, it is better for a mother to deliver spontaneously in the taxicab than go to a less-than-adequate hospital and have her baby held back by overwhelming sedatives or mechanical means. If the obstetrician suspects Rh problems, maternal diabetes, need for a Caesarean section, or likelihood of a premature birth, a pediatrician should be in attendance in the delivery room.

Bow LEGS   Most children look a little bow-legged when they start to walk. It does not represent rickets, which is rarely seen these days, but is rather a natural curving of the legs. Usually, after the child walks and grows—or by the time he gets beyond two years of age—his legs become more knock-kneed, and he looks flat-footed.

Grandmother's admonition not to let a baby walk too early is based on her fear of rickets, or soft bones. Nowadays, almost all milk contains vitamin D, and babies receive supplements of vitamin D along with other vitamins. If a baby wants to stand and he has been taking adequate doses of vitamin D, his bow-legged appearance is normal. It is frustrating to the baby to be hobbled so that he cannot walk. If he wants to walk early, it is perfectly all right to let him; if his back and legs bother him, he will stop walking and sit down.

BRAIN DAMAGE can be slight (which may result in a short attention span) or severe (as in the case of a prolonged coma or personality change after a stroke). Because nerves cannot regenerate like skin, any dead nerve is permanently lost; however, other parts of the vast brain complex may be able to assume the function of the damaged part. Slight insults to the brain are usually not detectable by electroencephalogram (EEG), neurological evaluation, or even inspection.

BREAST-FEEDING   A national group called La Leche League encourages mothers who are anxious to breast-feed their babies. I assume that most normal mothers want to attempt breast-feeding, but it is often difficult in many of our country's hospitals because there is no rooming-in procedure. However, because most mothers are discharged from the hospital in three to five days, and since milk does not really come in until the fourth day, the mother may still get home early enough to stimulate the production of breast milk, even if the hospital discouraged her. When faced with a brace of questions, a doctor's often-discouraging attitude is, "Forget it; try the bottle." Obviously, cow's milk is meant for calves, and human milk for babies. If you are equipped and motivated, you will probably be able to nurse your baby.

BREASTS IN BOYS between the ages of twelve and fifteen years are often tender and enlarged. This seems to be a common condition and does not mean that he is turning into a girl or is contracting cancer. Boys, of course, are terribly embarrassed, often refusing to ask about it, but are secretly very worried. The wise doctor will reassure the youth that the problem will go away, although it may take a year or so. Sometimes even light clothing will irritate the boy's nipples.

BREATH-HOLDING is usually a technique of the fifteen-month-old child who has rather severe and violent temper tantrums. He may hold his breath until he turns blue, his eyes roll, and he passes out. If this seems to be an almost daily routine, it might be wise to give the child a small amount of medication such as phenobarbital. This helps subdue his nervous system to the point that he will not pass out but will still have tantrums.

A mother who sees her child turning blue and becoming unconscious may overrespond to this distressing act, and because the child senses this means of getting extra attention, he may do it all the more. Small amounts of sedatives to abort the attacks might allow her to carry out her discipline in a more relaxed fashion.

CAROTENEMIA is a yellow discoloration of the skin fairly prominent in babies who are eating large amounts of yellow vegetables, such as carrots, squash, or sweet potatoes. It can be easily distinguished from jaundice, which gives a yellow tint to the whites of the eyes. In carotenemia, this yellow pigment is seen only in the skin, and is most obvious in the palms and soles of the feet. It is not serious, and usually implies that the child is on a reasonably good diet.

CEPHALOHEMATOMA is a rather alarming swelling on the head that appears in a significant number of babies shortly after birth. In the head's passage through the birth canal, a blood vessel underneath the scalp (but not under the skull) is broken, and the resulting hemorrhage makes a big bump, usually on the side of the head. It may or may not be associated with a fractured skull or deeper bleeding. In the old days, these lumps were thought to be devil's horns, and babies carrying them were thrown away! Formerly, doctors used to lance the scalp to remove the blood clot underneath, but too many babies developed infections. Doctors now treat cephalohematoma by leaving it alone; although the clot becomes encased in calcium. the swelling will eventually recede. After a year or two of life the baby will have a normal skull outline, although his mother can usually feel a little knobbiness on one side of the skull. In most cases it has nothing to do with the brain underneath and is strictly a reaction of the skull bone to injury, considered to be benign.

CEREBRAL PALSY is the general term for a wide variety of nerv- ous disorders, usually caused by birth trauma. In "scissors gait" the victim's legs are forced together so that it is difficult to put one foot ahead of the other. One arm may be held uselessly against the body, and usually becomes wasted because of lack of exercise.

CHOANAL STENOSIS is the narrowing of the nasal passageway where it joins the throat. The passageway may become small enough to trouble breathing when a new baby is nursing. Babies dislike breathing through their mouths, so they will become frantic and even blue; but as soon as they cry, their mouths open, and all seems normal. Diagnosis is made by passing a catheter through the nose.

CHOREA, or St. Vitus' Dance, is a rare neurological sign of rheu- matic fever. The victim is constantly writhing and twisting his arms, neck, and face muscles in a grotesque and purpose- less way; he is clumsy and spills things. The condition may be confused with a tic. (See Tics)

CIRCUMCISION has its advocates and detractors. Urologists tell us that they have never seen cancer of the penis in a circumcised male. The Jews started the practice, and at the time felt that it was a public-health measure. Circumcision now seems to be a national, cultural trait in the United States. Perhaps the only objection a pediatrician can bring is the possibility of the circumcised male developing an ammoniacal ulcer at the opening of the penis. Such ulcers can cause a stricture, which if not attended to can obstruct the flow of urine and put pres- sure on the bladder, and, if severe, this pressure can hurt the kidneys.

CLEFT PALATE is a birth defect in which the roof of the mouth has failed to form; it may be associated with a harelip. The internal structure of the nose can be seen through the mouth. The condition is associated with repeated ear infections. Plastic surgery repair is usually attempted by age eighteen months, so that speech will be distorted as little as possible. Since the operation often results in a shortened soft palate, the adenoids are not usually removed. This might increase the nasal quality of the child's speech.

CLOTHING should be adequate and comfortable. Many mothers have noticed that babies in the first few months of life have cold hands and feet. They bundle them up, assuming the children are cold or have some circulation problem. If a child weighs more than five or six pounds, he can probably be dressed in the same amount of clothing that is comfortable for other people in the household. If the room temperature is between 65° and 70° F. and if he is wearing a T-shirt, smock, and diapers plus bootees, he is probably adequately dressed.

Hands and feet are cold usually because most of the blood circulation is being directed to the intestines, where most of the body's work is progressing. A better way to tell a baby's general body temperature is to feel between his shoulder blades. If he is hot and sweaty there, then he is overdressed.

COLIC is any attack of stomach pain not due to hunger (see Chapter 2).

COLITIS is an inflammation of the colon that may be caused by a virus (as in the case of intestinal flu), a bacterium (as in bacillary dysentery, typhoid, or shigellosis that produces fever and bloody, foul-smelling stools), a parasite (amebic dysentery), an allergy (to milk or wheat), or unknown factors (ulcerative colitis). Treatment is rest, fluids, bland or white foods, and antibiotics if due to bacteria.

CONSTIPATION is the passage of hard, dry stools and has nothing to do with frequency of elimination. The consistency of the stool determines whether a person is or is not constipated. Obviously, people who have infrequent bowel movements tend to have harder ones, but some have normal stools once or twice a week. Some victims of constipation have their hard stools two or three times a day. Many constipated people feel sluggish, but not because they are absorbing poisons from the bacteria-laden stool resting in the colon. Most likely, the heavy stool itself and the extra blood supply the body is diverting to the lower intestine make the patient feel sluggish. Constipation does not lead to mental disorders. Occasionally, a child who is enjoying a fun-filled day does not have time to answer the call of nature. He will hold back his stool and as a result will become constipated.

Constipation is usually the result of eating too many white foods—milk, ice cream, cottage cheese, potatoes, bananas, applesauce, noodles, spaghetti, macaroni, bread, and other bakery goods. Because many children are on a dairy-product diet plus bread and rice and white foods, they are frequently constipated. You must make an effort to get your baby away from white foods exclusively.

If a child is still constipated after being put on a diet of meat, fruit, and vegetables, then try a safe laxative. Milk of magnesia is probably the best. Mineral oil may prevent the absorption of vitamins A and D into the system, and continuous ingestion may lead to bits of oil being deposited in the lungs, which appear as a spot in the X-ray.

CRADLE CAP is a collection of oily scales on the top of a baby's head. It is related to dandruff and can be a family trait. It is more likely to show up over the soft spot of the skull, since mothers are often reluctant to scrub at this area. They mistakenly feel that the brain is so close underneath this pulsating skin that they may push their finger through it.

If mild enough, various dandruff remedies are quite helpful in removing these scales. There is no cure for this, only control. Rubbing the scales with a mineral oil will usually soften them, and a subsequent bath with a soft brush and soap will remove them entirely. There are now special medicines that can be used, most of which contain sulfur, salicylic acid, or tar.

CRETIN is the name given to a congenitally hypothyroid dwarf. It is important to diagnose this condition early, since quick treatment with the thyroid hormone may prevent the mental retardation often associated with cretinism. The cretin baby is dry, cold, mottled, sluggish, usually constipated, and has a big tongue and prominent abdomen.

CRYPTORCHIDISM is the condition in which one or both testicles have not descended into the scrotum. Each year the urologists change their ground rules as to when they would like to operate to bring the undescended testicles down into the scrotum. At the present, between six and eight seems to be the recommended age. Most children are able to understand the need of an operation after they are six years of age, but this particular one should not be put off until adolescence. By that time, the testicle may have atrophied to the point that it will not function in adulthood.

CYSTIC FIBROSIS is a condition that is inherited as an autosomal recessive trait. Methods of control are more effective now than they were just a few years ago. There is no cure for this condition, but if properly treated, a patient can live a fairly normal life. Cystic fibrosis is manifested at birth by plugged intestines full of dry stool (no enzymes present.) Later, the infant has large, foul, bulky stools plus a bloated, gassy abdomen and thin arms, legs, and buttocks. Concurrent bronchitis, with much heavy green or yellow sputum, is the difficult part of the disease to control.

DEAFNESS   Parents are sometimes not aware of their deaf child's affliction until he is over eighteen months and has failed to utter an understandable word. Up to six months even a deaf baby will do some babbling, but if he cannot hear the approval of his parents, he will start making inhuman noises or just remain silent. A deaf baby will often watch his mother's lips instead of her eyes. Parents can make some attempt to test their child's hearing with suitable noisemakers in the first two months of life.

A doctor is sometimes unable to diagnose congenital or nerve deafness because the eardums appear perfectly normal. It is important to recognize congenital deafness because of the need for early treatment. If a child has normal speech, he was born able to hear. But when he gets to be four or five and has been afflicted with a number of ear infections, he may develop deafness in one ear that may go undetected since his speech is normal. Children's ears and hearing should be checked periodically. Sometimes simple tests at home will suffice, such as whispering to a child while plugging one ear with your finger. Do not let your child see your lips move while you test him. Of course, a more scientific audiogram in the doctor's office is mandatory if you have any suspicions of a real problem.

DEATH If a loved one dies, children should be informed of the situation in an honest way. Questions should be answered directly and immediately. Parents should not try to hide their grief from a child, who should see them laugh when they are happy and cry when they are sad. In this way, they learn appropriate emotions for different situations.

CRIB DEATHS Small babies, usually between three months and a year of age, who die suddenly in their crib at night have stimulated a great deal of investigation. A mother should realize that a baby does not suffocate if he has the least ability to move his head around. An infant sleeping under the blanket or face down on the sheet does not suffocate all by himself. Some doctors believe crib death is due to some strange hormone or parathyroid malfunction; others, that it is an overwhelming virus infection to which the baby has built up no immunity. (Indeed, some of these babies have been found to have low amounts of gamma globulin and thus little power to fight off overwhelming infections.) Another theory is that in a certain number of cases, the baby has had a milk allergy. Two or three drops of milk have come up from the stomach and lodged in the bronchial tubes, causing an overwhelming allergic spasm and, of course, death. Present research should soon give some answers.

DEHYDRATION usually follows fever, vomiting, or diarrhea. So much fluid and minerals have left the baby's system that he usually goes into a state of acidosis. If a child has intestinal flu with the above symptoms and still is able to sit up, move around, and urinate two or three times a day, he is not so severely dehydrated that he needs to be hospitalized and receive intravenous fluids. However, you should forestall his problem lest it become severe or irreversible. A new suppository containing tranquilizers has proved greatly beneficial to children suffering from the vomiting of twenty-four-hour flu. Most babies can tolerate a few hours of vomiting, after which you should seek a doctor's prescription for this type of anti-emetic. Usually it slows down the vomiting enough so that the baby does not lose too much stomach fluid and may even be able to take sips of juice, broth, or water. But if the patient is listless and his skin has lost its normal elastic quality, he is in trouble. Usually minerals are lost with water and must be replaced simultaneously. Cola and other soft drinks—rather than plain water—are better to offer the vomiting child.

DEVIL'S GRIP is the inflammation of the diaphragm muscle and is caused by a virus. The result is pain in the region of the entire lower rib cage during inspiration and it may be confused with pleurisy.

DOWN'S SYNDROME is a more fitting name for what was formerly called mongolism. It occurs about once in every seven hundred births, most frequently to the children of women near the end of their child-bearing years, and is believed to be a chromosomal abnormality in almost all cases. All afflicted babies are mentally defective and have relaxed musculature. There is usually a flatness to the back of the head, an epicanthic fold of the eyelids, short fingers, and other signs that, taken together, make diagnosis simple. A baby with this problem changes its family's whole pattern of living, and the emotional impact of course falls most heavily on the mother. She must be given as much information about the condition as possible before deciding what is best for her and her family. She may listen but not necessarily accept advice from well-meaning friends, neighbors, or relatives. Some mothers find it most appropriate to have the baby institutionalized; others may decide to keep the child. Once the decision is made, her family, her doctor, her relatives, and her friends must back her up completely.

DWARFISM is generally defined as a lack of, or slow, growth. In the first year of life, a baby grows close to nine or ten inches; in the second year, three or four inches. Between the age of five to the onset of puberty, the average growth rate is two to three inches a year. Slower development implies there may be some interference with the growth process, possibly due to chronic heart or kidney disease. The possibility of thyroid hypofunction is next on the list. Dwarfism due to the lack of pituitary growth hormone is very rare. Various tests can determine the cause, and specific measures can be instituted for some types. Continuous observation of a child is the most important way to spot this rather serious defect early in life.

ECZEMA is a rash characterized by redness, scaliness, itchiness, and in most cases, a weepy surface. In about half of the cases, some definite link can be established with a food allergy. If a complete change of diet has no real effect on the eczema, the problem is called atopic. Various medicines, soaps, and ointments can be used to control the condition, which becomes much milder after the age of eighteen months. Most eczema victims will grow up to have other allergic manifestations such as hay fever or asthma. The only treatment is control.

ELECTROENCEPHALOGRAM (EEG) is an ink tracing of the amplified brain waves picked up by sensitive wires placed on the skull. It can be helpful in diagnosing problems such as brain tumors, blood clots, and epilepsy. At one time it was hoped that peculiar behavior and abnormal brain waves could be correlated, but much research has indicated that the EEG is not infallible. For instance, not every patient with epilepsy will show an abnormal EEG. An estimated 10 to 15 percent of apparently normal people with no nervous symptoms demonstrate abnormal brain waves.

ENCOPRESIS is the passage of small amounts of stool into the patient's underwear, either consciously or unconsciously. This is occasionally a physical or organic problem related to constipation, diarrhea, colitis, or allergies; but is most often a sign of subconscious aggression. The patient is apparently venting his hostility through this socially unaccepted form. A certain amount of encopresis is normal up to three or four years of age. But beyond the age of five or six, it is usually a symptom serious enough to require constructive psychological care.

EPILEPSY is a general term for a seizure originating from the nervous system. It may manifest itself by a generalized convulsion, by staring into space, or by visceral or autonomic reactions. Some headaches and stomachaches can be a form of epilepsy, although the term usually refers to attacks in which the patient temporarily loses consciousness. Epilepsy may be chemical or physical in origin, but in a vast majority of cases the cause is unknown. Usually an electroencephalogram (EEG) is diagnostic. Medicines such as Dilantin and phenobarbital are effective controls.

EPINEPHRINE (adrenalin) is a chemical secreted by the adrenal glands which prepare the body for fight or flight. When injected it stimulates the heart to beat faster, but it is mainly used for the relief of asthma. It may be life-saving in severe allergic reactions, such as bee stings or laryngeal spasm due to food allergies.

EYES

Plugged tear duct. Perhaps one out of every ten babies is born with mucus plugging the canal that runs from the inner corner of the eye into the nose carrying tears from the eyes into the nasal passage. If the duct is plugged with mucus, tears cannot flow properly. This may cause infection, in which case green or yellow material forms in the eyes and may cause the lids to stick together. The condition usually disappears in the first three to six months, but the ducts can be helped by gently massaging the area on the side of the nose just below the inner corner of the eye. Infections can usually be controlled by suitable sulfa or antibiotic eye drops or ointment. In any case, the problem is not serious and does not damage vision.

Cross-eyes, strabismus, or squint is the inability of the eyes to focus and work together. Most babies have some difficulty using binocular vision until they are six months old, but if their eyes do not move together after this age, ophthalmological consultation is necessary. However, the eye people have trouble curing this difficulty with glasses or surgery, and most pediatricians make the mistake of sending babies to the eye doctor either too early or too late. You should make an effort to evaluate vision in each eye early in life. What appears to be cross-eyes often results from a mere flattening of the bridge of the nose, which allows the skin to overlap the inner aspect of each eyeball. If a baby truly has cross-eyes or wall-eyes, he will learn to use just one eye and will ignore the image that comes from the other, resulting in a condition known as amblyopia.

Amblyopia is blindness or defective vision in an eye. If good binocular vision is not established in a cross-eyed child by the time he is four or five, this suppressive blindness can be permanent.

Glaucoma is an abnormal accumulation of fluid inside the eye that leads to increased pressure. In a baby this sometimes can be detected by feeling the eyes through the closed lids. In some patients, the first symptom is an enlarged pupil and a misty cornea. An operation can often solve the problem.

FEET AND LEGS

Flat feet. Until the age of four or five, most children are quite flat-footed. Contrary to the feelings of shoe salesmen, it is not necessary to provide them with stiff shoes for arch support. A child's foot will usually develop an arch by the time he is six years old, but if his genes say that he is going to have flat feet, he is going to have flat feet. Arch supports usually do nothing but raise the arch temporarily, and when the lifts are removed the arches flop down again. Picking up marbles with the toes does not help develop an arch or a good working foot. However, I would assume that running barefoot over wet sand at the beach or over clods of dirt or soft turf might help develop the smaller muscles of the arch.

The pigeon-toed child usually had his feet and legs crossed over his abdomen when he was in the uterus. After birth, he slept on his stomach in the knee-chest position, with his toes turned inward, which only aggravated the pigeon-toed tendency. The condition is usually associated with a so-called tibial torsion, in which the shin bone spirals between the knee and the foot. A doctor's assessment is usually necessary, because the early use of splints or braces may correct pigeon toes during the period of rapid growth.

The knock-kneed child is almost universally seen between the ages of two and four. When standing at what may be called "attention" with his knees barely touching, a normal child usually has two to three inches of space between his ankle bones. If there is more than five inches of space between his ankle bones, you might consider the use of an inner heel or sole wedge, which serves to push the knees out by raising up the inner border of the foot. If you and your husband are extremely knock-kneed, your child may inherit the same trait. However, most children who go barefoot or only wear tennis shoes will largely outgrow the knock-kneed tendency by the time they are six or seven.

The dislocated hip is sometimes difficult to discover until the child begins to walk, even though the doctor may have made the proper search for this not uncommon tendency. The hip may have been in a position of partial dislocation, and dislocate completely only when forced to bear weight. Because his hip joint is not stable when the child takes a step, he has to tip his body to the side of the affected hip in a rather grotesque way, thus giving away his problem. Treatment is much simpler if the condition is discovered in early infancy. Make sure your doctor has done the dislocated-hip test at least once.

FISTULA is an abnormal tunnel connecting one organ to another or one organ to the skin. For example, the appendix may burst and after surgical removal of the pus, fecal matter may drain from the large bowel, through the appendix remnant to the outside.

FLUORIDE is a chemical naturally found in the soil, and thus also in the drinking water in a large part of the world. In trace amounts, the element is necessary for the proper structure of teeth and bones. If provided in the proper amounts in the first eight years of a child's life, it can delay tooth decay and may even reduce the bone demineralization suffered by older people. Most health authorities now believe that fluoride should be added to the community water. If this is impossible, families should get a prescription for it so they can give proper amounts to their growing children. Fluoridation is not a Communist plot, nor does it soften the brain or harden the kidneys.

FOOD is obviously necessary for life. During infancy, milk is perhaps the most important food, but after the first ten months of life—and especially from the age of one year on—milk is to be discouraged and meat and fruit encouraged. Most children dislike vegetables, but fruit and vegetables are quite interchangeable. Probably the best diet includes generous portions of meats, fruits, and grains, and maybe some dairy products. A mother in doubt as to the proper foods to feed her child should remember that meat and fruit are probably the most important ones. White foods such as carbohydrates and potatoes, noodles and spaghetti, should be used as extras to satisfy energy requirements, but the basic meat and fruit should be provided almost daily.

GAMMA GLOBULIN is one of the blood proteins. Blood protein fractions are named according to their molecular size. The gamma—or largest size protein—of the globulin is assumed to be the storehouse of the antibodies or disease-fighting protein. It is the portion that prevents a person from suffering more than once from measles, chicken pox, mumps, and polio. Some people are naturally deficient in their gamma globulin and are subject to serious and often overwhelming infections. If your child is sickly and frequently develops high fevers, pneumonias, abscessed ears, or tonsillitis, it is worth checking the level of gamma globulin in his blood.

HEART MURMURS are sounds heard between the two beats of the heart. The main beats heard through the stethoscope are the closing of various valves, and murmurs heard in between can arise from a variety of conditions. The organic heart murmur is due to specific defects in which the blood seeps through incompetent valves or through the walls separating the heart chambers. Functional murmurs imply that the heart is basically sound, but basically noisy. Certain vibrations of the various cords and walls can create murmurs, as can the whirlpool effect of blood going rapidly from one chamber to another. An estimated one out of every three children has a functional heart murmur. It means nothing, except that a doctor may misinterpret it and cause a family needless concern.

HEMANGIOMA is the "strawberry birthmark." It usually enlarges until its wearer is one year of age, at which time it begins to recede. It becomes dull red, and small areas begin to bleach out as the capillaries become obliterated. It leaves an area of thin skin that does not tan well; but if allowed to disappear spontaneously, there is less of a scar than if dry ice or X rays are used to hurry it away. Watchful waiting is the best treatment.

HERNIA is the bulging produced when any organ protrudes through a weakness in the muscle walls that are supposed to hold it in place. Usually the offending organ is a loop of intestine that pushes through an abdominal muscle. The navel or umbilical hernia is *not* due to improper care at birth, but due to slow closure of the hole through which the baby has been nourished before birth. The squishy loop of bowel that sticks out appears about to burst—but it does not. As the baby grows, the tissues about the navel firm up, sealing off the opening. Taping and/or surgery are not necessary.

The *inguinal* hernia is common in the male. The sperm tube from the testicle goes through the abdominal muscles just above and to the side of the pubic bone, and if this opening is a little too big, slight straining or crying will urge a loop of intestine through it and down into the scrotum. You may notice the swelling that comes and goes, and thus make the diagnosis better than your doctor can (who may only be able to detect a slightly enlarged inguinal "ring"). Surgery is necessary for the inguinal hernia, since if the intestine ever gets stuck in the scrotum, an emergency operation will be required.

HIVES, an allergic skin reaction, are blotchy, often very extensive patches of red, slightly raised, itchy skin. They appear a few minutes to a few hours after the victim has ingested some food to which he is sensitive. Once the reaction has appeared, it may continue for hours or days, cropping out in different areas. Soda baths, antihistamines, and ointments may help the patient live through his distress; only rarely does a severe case need cortisone. It is possible to pinpoint the cause of hives in only about half the cases, although strawberries, tomatoes, citrus fruits, chocolates, and nuts are the most likely offenders.

HYDROCELE is a collection of a waterlike fluid in the space

around the testicle. It is common in small boys, but almost always disappears by itself by one or two years of age. This condition is occasionally associated with and/or confused with a scrotal hernia.

HYDROCEPHALUS is "water on the brain," an excess accumulation of the spinal fluid normally found in and around the brain. Causes are largely unknown. The building pressure of the liquid separates the thin skull bones of an infant, and if allowed to continue, will destroy brain tissue. Ingenious neurosurgical shunts have been devised to drain off the fluid before damage occurs.

HYPOSPADIAS is a condition in which the male urethra (the tube carrying urine from the bladder to the end of the penis) ends short of its normal exit. The opening can be found anywhere from just behind the head of the penis to the region of the scrotum. If its position precludes normal urinary or ejaculatory functions, surgery is required to straighten out the plumbing and save the victim from inconvenience and embarrassment.

IMMUNIZATIONS, now routine, are vaccines of weakened or dead bacteria that help the body develop the proper antibodies to fight off infections. The system can practice getting rid of "de-fanged" germs before the real thing comes along. The DPT shots (Diphtheria—Pertussis (whooping cough)—Tetanus) are traditionally given together in the first few months. Three separate injections are needed. DPT booster shots are standard procedure at eighteen to twenty-four months and at five to six years. After age six, just D-T is administered routinely every ten years. If a year has elapsed from the last booster, another should be given following a puncture wound.

The triple Salk killed-polio vaccine (injection) or the Sabin live-polio vaccine (oral) may be given at the same time as the DPT. Smallpox vaccinations are best given after ten months, but before eighteen months, unless there is an active case of eczema in the home. Polio and smallpox boosters should be given at least every ten years.

Live-measles vaccine is given at twelve months. Live-mumps vaccine is new, safe, and especially important to give to males before maturity.

Typhoid, cholera, yellow fever, and typhus immunizations are necessary before entering areas known to harbor these illnesses.

Gamma globulin will provide passive immunity to hepatitis and measles. It will make chicken pox a little easier for a baby who has been exposed to an older sibling. Repeated smallpox vaccinations can cut down the frequency of recurrent canker sores. Some doctors have success giving a series of dead staphylococcus bacteria injections to people suffering from frequent boils, sties, and skin infections. Also, a few injections of a vaccine made up of dead bacteria usually found in the respiratory passages can minimize sinus and bronchial infections.

INTESTINAL OBSTRUCTIONS can occur anywhere in the twenty-odd feet of bowel between the stomach and the rectum. If the anal opening is not present (*atresia*), vomiting and cramps begin at birth. *Anal stenosis* (narrowing) does not produce vomiting until the bowels become overdistended with food and gas. *Pyloric stenosis* (see Section II) produces symptoms in the first six weeks. *Intussusception* (telescoping of one part of the bowel into another) and *volvulus* (knotting or twisting of a bowel segment around itself) usually produce excruciating, colicky pain, and vomiting. *Megacolon* (an absence of the nerves that stimulate the bowel wall muscles to push stools through the lower colon) produces obstinate constipation and an enlarged abdomen requiring enemata.

All of these conditions require the attention of a surgeon—some immediately, some after proper preparatory treatment.

IPECAC SYRUP is a powerful emetic. It is well worth having in the medicine closet for the rare (I hope) occasion when your child ingests poison. The two- to three-year-old is most likely to be less than a gourmet in his selection of things to swallow. If so, three teaspoons of this syrup usually induces copious vomiting in about fifteen to twenty minutes. Vomiting empties the stomach more efficiently than pumping, but the latter technique may be required if the ipecac does not work. Kerosene, gasoline, and other volatile hydrocarbons, if vomited, may trickle into the lungs and set up a severe chemical pneumonia. (See "Poisonings" in Section I.)

IRON is the metallic ion found in the hemoglobin molecule. Iron deficiency accounts for the anemia seen most often in children who live on milk to the exclusion of meat and fruits or vegetables. White foods are poor sources of iron. Those who are pale, weak, tired, or sick due to anemia, may need an iron tonic.

JAUNDICE is a yellow tinge showing in the whites of eyes and skin. It is a symptom of several diseases, the most common one being hepatitis. A baby with erythroblastosis turns yellow-orange because of the rapid destruction of his red blood cells. A high level of this bilirubin pigment can damage a newborn baby's brain, but an exchange transfusion of blood will wash this pigment out of his system before a dangerous level is reached.

KETOSIS is the accumulation of ketone chemicals in the blood. It occurs during dehydration, malnutrition, acidosis, and cyclic vomiting—whenever the body is forced to draw on stored fats for energy. The victim's breath has a fruity smell; a simple urine test is the clincher.

LEAD is a heavy metal which, if ingested, can cause poisoning. Lead-free paint should be used on furniture and toys. Lead intoxication can come from breathing the air in polluted industrial areas or in homes where lead batteries are burned as fuel.

LYMPH GLANDS or nodes, found all over the body, act as traps that collect debris and neutralize local infections. The nodes that most commonly give trouble are those high in the neck, directly under the corners of the jawbone. In strep or sore throats these usually swell and become tender, and enlarge in infectious mononucleosis. Virus infections such as roseola and chicken pox swell the glands on the back of the head and neck. An infection in the hand or arm can cause the armpit glands to swell; the glands in the groin will similarly enlarge from an infected toe or skinned knee. Cat-scratch disease is not uncommon and will cause regional nodes to enlarge in various places. Any glands that swell without a local infection to explain them should be investigated, since this is (only rarely, though) a sign of cancer or leukemia.

MASTURBATION is the autostimulation of the genital area to produce pleasurable sensations or orgasm. It is so common in male adolescents that if a boy does not do it, he may be abnormal. Only 40 to 50 percent of females practice it. In no way does it lead to mental derangement, laziness, or pimples. Parents must never create guilt feelings in their child about masturbation, since it is not a problem and is a sign of health.

Most three- to seven-year-old children discover this exciting area but will disregard it unless a case of allergy, a fungus, or worms serves to draw their attention to it. Rarely, an emotionally ill child may use this easy gratification as a substitute for more rewarding social contacts.

MEGACOLON is an enlarged colon usually produced by a narrow segment of non-functioning intestine near the rectum. The nearby colon becomes distended with gas and stool and requires enemata from early infancy to deflate it. Surgery is necessary to remove the defective area.

MENSTRUATION is the passage of the endometrium (lining of the uterus) every twenty to thirty days in the female if conception fails to occur. The menarche, the first menstruation, signals the end of puberty at the average age of twelve or thirteen. The girl is now a woman, but she may not yet be fertile, as her ovaries may not be producing eggs. She usually requires two years for her periods to become regular. Growth slows after this first period, and no more than one or two inches is added. Menstrual pain requiring codeine and bed rest may need investigation. The flow usually continues for three to five days; it is appropriate to use a comfortable tampon which will not jeopardize the girl's virginal status. Temporary interruption of menstrual regularity (amenorrhea) may follow sickness, emotional upset, or malnutrition, though pregnancy is still the most common cause.

MIGRAINE can be diagnosed in children age five to ten, providing the headaches are episodic and the family has a history of this condition. A child's first symptom may be cyclic vomiting; as time goes on, the vomiting diminishes and the headaches worsen. The headache may be all over, not just on one side, and may or may not produce spots in front of eyes or flashes of light. Some children show ketone substances in their urine the day before an attack; medicine given at that time will occasionally abort the onset.

Victims of migraine often tend to be tense, quick, driven people—they are built this way, and their headaches are a part of their personality. It is not an emotional or psychiatric disease, although tension does aggravate the symptoms.

MONGOLISM—see Down's Syndrome.

MONGOLOID SPOTS are blue, irregular areas resembling bruises found over the sacral region of Oriental babies. They may also appear on Indians or on babies of Mediterranean origin. They fade with age.

NEVI or moles are the brown pigmented spots most of us have sprinkled over our body. Someone who bothered to count them found the average adult has about forty. Doctors used to be taught to remove nevi on the hands, feet, and genitalia, as these were thought more likely to become malignant. If you note a change in the color or size of a mole, or if itching or bleeding occurs, removal is a good idea. In general, removal is recommended for any skin tumor or growth that is not clearly benign.

OBESITY means excess weight. The standard height and weight charts in most doctor's offices are now considered obsolete— if you look fat, you are. Researchers now feel that many psychological, neurological, hormonal, and genetic factors are responsible for overweight, besides habit and exercise. The fat child eats without feeling full, as if his calories went directly from stomach to fat-storage depots without letting his brain know what happened in between. The fat child often becomes the fat adult, but *not* necessarily because his mother stuffed him. She may try to feed him less, but he will steal the food when hunger overwhelms him. (When he is an adolescent, he will blame her for not trying harder to make him thin.) Motivation is the key to losing weight—until research finds the hormone or enzyme fault responsible.

OSGOOD-SCHLATTER'S DISEASE is an irritation of the growing (top) end of the tibia or shinbone. It occurs between the ages of nine to eleven years, and produces a dull aching knob about an inch below the kneecap that may last as long as twelve months. The pain disappears, but the extra calcium deposit may be permanent.

PHOBIA is the Latin word for fear. School phobia is the most common one in the growing child. Fear of the unknown is less likely to make the child panic at the thought of going to school—more likely his worry is that his parents will disappear or the home will break up if he leaves. In any event, it is imperative to get him to go, since the longer he is out, the harder it is for him to return. Some type of psychotherapy may also be necessary.

PICA is the persistent eating of nonfood items, especially dirt. It suggests malnutrition, or at least anemia.

PILONIDAL DIMPLE is a common small depression or pit found at the base of the spine. With irritation it may become infected, occasionally appearing as a tender boil. Permanent cure requires surgery.

PUBERTY is the period during which a child matures physically and sexually. Rapid growth occurs and secondary sexual characteristics appear. Moodiness, depression, stubbornness, fatigue, clumsiness, and rebellion are common—requiring sympathy, patience, and reasonable rules from parents.

RASH is defined as any redness, scale, blister, papule, or pimple that develops suddenly. You should use the proper names when describing a rash to a doctor: a *macule* is a flat red area; a *papule* is a raised area. A drop of clear fluid in a papule is a *vesicle*. A larger vesicle is a blister. A *pustule* is a blister filled with yellow or green pus. If the top layer is off, it is an *excoriation*. The measles rash, for example, is macular. Chicken pox is maculopapular becoming vesicular, then pustular, then crusted.

Redness about the anal area or between the buttocks is usually dietary or allergic in origin. Peaches and citrus are common causes. Vesicles and blisters forming where urine is in contact with the skin usually result from an ammonia burn. Papules becoming pustular on the buttocks are most frequently due to chocolate ingestion. Eczema is red and scaly and very itchy, like most allergic rashes. A very solid red rash over the genitalia with a sharp border of small vesicles is usually thrush (see "Monilia" in Section II), most often seen in the newborn if the mother has had vaginal moniliasis (yeast infection) in the latter days of her pregnancy.

A *contact* rash is usually red and scaly. If it occurs on the neck, the cause may be a plastic bib; in the diaper area, rubber pants; on the feet, nylon stockings or plastic shoe inserts; on the hands, wool gloves.

SPINAL TAP or puncture is the diagnostic needling of the space about the spinal cord. The spinal fluid flowing in this area will be carrying pus cells in the case of meningitis, lymph cells in the cases of polio, or mumps encephalitis, or blood after a severe head injury or stroke. It is a valuable test, it is safe, and should be agreed to if your doctor suggests it.

SPLEEN is a mysterious lymphatic organ found behind the lower left rib area. Its enlargement suggests a number of diseases, from mononucleosis to leukemia. When enlarged and injured, it may hemorrhage severely and require surgical removal.

TESTES, or testicles, are normally found in the scrotum at birth. They have descended from within the body during the prenatal months. If only one is present, its undescended mate should be brought down into the scrotum surgically at about age six to eight years. Otherwise, it may atrophy and be functionless. If *both* are undescended, they may come down of their own accord at puberty; however, a hormone test should be attempted early to see whether they will be responsive at that later time.

THYMUS is a gland full of lymph tissue, found just behind the upper part of the breastbone. It is important for disease immunity, especially in the young infant, and was once erroneously thought to be the cause of sudden crib deaths.

THYROID GLAND secretes a hormone responsible for metabolism and growth. A *hypo*thyroid condition is the result of less than adequate amounts of hormone, and is fairly easy to detect in a child because of his failure to grow at least two inches a year. If in addition to a slow growth rate the child is sluggish, has dry, cold skin, and is constipated, he is probably hypothyroid. The *hyper*thyroid condition (too much hormone) is very rare in childhood and may be confused with the hypermotor child. Blood tests for thyroxine are quite accurate as an aid to the diagnosis. A fat, warm, pink-cheeked child who perspires easily almost surely does not have a hypothyroid problem. Goitre is a soft, swollen thyroid gland usually found in people whose diets have been low in iodine.

TICS are isolated muscle spasms, but may also be broadly defined to include integrated reactions of the whole body. A few tics are so violent and episodic as to suggest convulsions, and most of these are family-related. The more attention you pay to them, the more they seem to crop up.

  Bed-rocking is a noisy, rhythmical, whole body motion that many infants need to go through to initiate sleep—like a dog turning around three times. Placing the mattress on the floor may prevent damage of furniture, walls, and floor. The habit stops when the need to rock has been dissipated, and that is that. Punishment will only increase frustration for both child and parent.

  Head-banging is like bed-rocking. The calcium deposit that forms at the site of trauma soon disappears when the banging does. No known brain damage seems to develop from this distressing habit—it only serves to drive parents wild.

Thumb-sucking is more common in colicky babies. Once it is established it is usually too late to substitute the pacifier, (the Nuk is best), which has less of a tendency to create malaligned teeth. If you look on thumb-sucking as a normal infantile phase, your child will be more likely to abandon it between two to five years of age.

Nail-biting is frequently associated with advanced thumb-suckers who seem to need this oral pleasure. You cannot stop this unless you provide a substitute, pleasurable function. Most children will cease this habit because their friends think it is immature and *not* because their mother said to do so.

TOILET-TRAINING ties more parents into psychological knots than any other area of child-rearing. Learning waits on maturation; when the child feels it is time to use the toilet, he will. After all, it is a fairly complicated act—the child has to be able to relax some muscles and contract others. Girls usually train themselves at two years and boys at three years. The longer you wait before pointing to the toilet, the shorter the training period will be. If you use the toilet, so will your child. Some parents will send their untrained three-year-old to nursery school, telling the teacher he *is* trained; and sometimes the ploy will work. At potty time, he will cheerfully go because all the others are doing it and he wants to be accepted.

TONGUE-TIE is not a cause of speech impediment unless the frenum under the tongue is so thick and short that the tongue is immobile (this is rare). Clipping the short, thick membrane will at least release the psychological tension of some parents who believe that speech problems and tongue-tie are related.

Geography tongue is the map-like configuration of tongue papillae. At one time it was believed that patterns on the tongue were a manifestation of internal disease.

TONSILLECTOMY (see "Adenoids") is the surgical removal of the tonsils and is associated with some risk. Size is not the main factor for removal. You should consider the operation, however, if repeated tonsil infections occur after age six or seven.

(more than two or three a year) and the glands in the neck stay swollen between attacks.

ULCERS of the duodenum are usually assumed to occur only in tense, nervous, worried, compulsive adults; hence, they often go undiagnosed in childhood. Many children are constitutionally rigid and self-demanding with high achievement goals; ulcers seem to be a part of their personality. Epigastric pain on an empty stomach, which is relieved by food or antacids, is a giveaway—especially if there are other ulcer victims in the family. In such a case, an X ray (barium meal) would at least reveal an "irritable duodenum" if it did not show an actual ulcer.

UMBILICUS is the scientific name for navel or belly button (see "Hernia"). It is perfectly safe to bathe a newborn baby whose cord remnant is still attached. The soap, water, and alcohol used may dry the stump and slight bleeding may occur. After the bath, it is wise to tease a dollop of antibiotic ointment onto the area where the skin and stump join. When the cord has separated, continual use of this ointment on the raw umbilical wound may prevent dryness, bleeding, and secondary infection.

URETER is the narrow tube which carries urine from the kidney to the bladder. It is the frequent site of anomalies which prevent the free flow of urine and can result in subsequent pyelitis and kidney damage.

URETHRA is the tube which carries urine from the bladder to the outside. Because it is short in the female, bacteria migrate more easily up into the bladder to produce cystitis or at least pus in the urine. The circumcised male infant frequently gets an ulcer just at or inside the urethral opening at the end of the penis from an ammonia burn. If untreated, this opening could scar or narrow and produce a back pressure of urine into bladder and kidneys.

VIRUS is the term given to an ultramicroscopic particle which multiplies inside the body cells and produces various disease states: measles, flu, mumps, chicken pox, colds, canker sores, polio, etc. Specific anti-viral agents have not yet proved as effective as have antibiotics against bacterial infections. A specific virus is responsible for a specific disease, although infection by one may produce immunity against another: previous infection by the cowpox virus (vaccination) will protect the body from smallpox (and sometimes the canker sore virus). Most children have about forty to sixty different virus infections before age seven, at which time they normally have only one or two a year (one or two bad colds a year, one attack of vomiting and diarrhea every year or so, one attack of fever and laryngeal cough every two or three years). Eighty percent of children's infections are "the virus that is going around."

Vitamins

Vitamin A is found in butter, milk, eggs, and yellow vegetables. Deficiency leads to visual problems and dry skin. Carefully supervised large doses administered for short periods of time will improve some acne and eczema conditions. Vitamin A in overdoses acts as a poison.

Vitamin B is found in grain and meat. Deficiency leads to weakness, neuritis, and skin and bowel problems. A good general diet provides satisfactory amounts, and an overdose is a waste. Some people find they are less frequently bitten by mosquitoes when taking B_1, or B complex vitamins, or brewers' yeast.

Vitamin C is found in fresh fruits. Deficiency leads to scurvy, bleeding gums, and easy bruising. Again, excess is a waste and will not prevent colds.

Vitamin D is synthesized by the skin whenever it is exposed to sunshine or even blue sky. It is also found in some milk and butter. Any excess is stored in the body and may become poisonous. Vitamin D appears to aid the absorption of calcium from the intestines and its deposit into teeth and bones. Deficiency leads to rickets or soft bones.

Vitamin E is probably essential to metabolism, but not all is known about its use in the body.

Vomiting is the rejection of stomach and/or intestinal contents (see "Obstruction"). This return of food may be due to (1) not enough room (obstruction, overfeeding, swallowed air), (2) allergy (usually to cow's milk), (3) fat intolerance, or (4) disease (intestinal flu, tonsillitis, kidney infection, meningitis, acidosis). Several types are listed, in order of severity:

Spit or *wet burp*, (two to fou. easpoons of vomit), *urp*, (one to two tablespoons), *emesis*, (two to six ounces), *vomitus*, (four to eight ounces with force), *heaves*, (six to eight ounces with great force), *projectile emesis*, (a large amount violently shot out two to three feet from the victim). The latter two types are more likely to be associated with an obstruction. Passage of bile, feces, or coffee-ground emesis (blood) is serious.

WARTS are now considered to be caused by the skin's reaction to a virus (not to dirt or to handling frogs). After months or years the usual ones on the hands may disappear spontaneously. When they appear on the bottom of the feet (the plantar area) they are called plantar warts. Because of the discomfort they produce, they are usually removed by surgery or chemical applications. X-ray is now used less frequently.

WITCH'S MILK is a thin milky secretion which comes from a baby's engorged breasts at birth due to the influence of the mother's lactogenic hormone. If breast-fed, the baby retains the condition for several weeks. Poking or squeezing the breasts will only irritate them and may cause an infection.

INDEX

A

Abcesses, 148, 166-67
Abdomen, areas of, 182
Accidents, 157
Acetone, 183
Achondroplasia, 183
Acidosis, 183
Acne, 183
Addison's disease, 183-84
Adenoids, 185
Adoption, 184
  hypermotor children and, 84
Adrenalin, *See* Epinephrine
Albuminuria, 185
Allergies, 4, 6, 107-22, 185
  appearance as psychosomatic
    problems of, 107-110
  of babies, 113-14
  bed-wetting caused by, 70-71
  colds caused by, 115-17

contactants most likely to cause,
  120
foods most likely to cause, 119
headaches caused by, 9, 111-12
inhalation, 117-18
most likely causes, 120
preparation of dust-free room to
    alleviate, 121-22
to milk, 6, 111-12, 113
  bottle feeding and, 21-22, 23
  breast feeding and, 15, 17
to one's own bacteria, 115-17
  medication for, 116
psychological problems resulting
    from, 118-19
sleep problems caused by, 64
symptoms of, 111-13
  nasal, 112, 146
  urinary, 112
to vitamins, 109-110
Alopecia, 185